Dance Like Nobody's Watching

By

Marion Rosen

Copyright © 2002 by Marion Rosen

ISBN 0-7414-1199-7

Cover art by Ellen Rosen and Natalie Rosen

Published by:

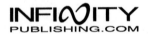
PUBLISHING.COM

519 West Lancaster Avenue
Haverford, PA 19041-1413
Info@buybooksontheweb.com
www.buybooksontheweb.com
Toll-free (877) BUY BOOK
Local Phone (610) 520-2500
Fax (610) 519-0261

Printed in the United States of America

Printed on Recycled Paper

Published August, 2002

I dedicate this book:

To the memory of those brave warriors who fought the good fight but lost the battle nonetheless:

Maria N. Alvarez
Barbara Foerster
Tina Louise Rollo
Virginia Benson
Grace Hinnershitz
Marge Brinkworth
Irene Woolley

To all the courageous cancer survivors I've met over the years at The Wellness Community and to the caring staff members who touched my heart:

Anne Gessert
Maryana Palmer
Marty Nason
Toni Feld Parker

To all my other cancer "buddies" who gave me support and hope:

Blandette Bush
Linda Blaustein
Toni Domenic
Patricia Klein
Maureen "Corky" Burrill

To Dr. Janice A. Schilling, Dr. Edward Chang, and Dr. Neal Semrad who got me through the worst and to Dr. Jia-ling Chou and Dr. Scott Sanborn for continued guidance.

To my friend Ruth Baker for organizing meals on wheels to feed my family and for providing countless hours of telephone therapy to feed my soul.

To my sister and her husband, Betty and John Morrisson, for listening and actually hearing, a true act of love.

And finally to those who most of all continue to love and support me:

My husband and best friend Morrie Rosen.
My son Scott Rosen, his wife Ellen Rosen
and their children Natalie and Ryan Rosen.
My daughter and my own special nurse, Nancy De Channes
and her daughter Madeleine "Maddie" De Channes.
My daughter Deborah Kiel, her husband Barnett Kiel
and their daughters Briana and Lyla Kiel.

SPECIAL THANKS TO:

My daughter-in-law, Ellen Rosen, for designing the cover of this book, and to my granddaughter, Natalie Rosen, age 7, for her wonderfully creative and meticulous artwork.

My son Scott Rosen and Ruth's son, Jonathan Baker, for their patience in helping me to overcome my computer "illiteracy."

And finally my deepest gratitude to Linda Ruhle, my healer, for her wisdom, guidance, and love.

DANCE LIKE NOBODY'S WATCHING

Cancer

When I received a phone call from my HMO telling me that my recent mammogram was inconclusive, I didn't panic. Breast cancer did not run in my family, so the vague, irregular density they had detected in my right breast was probably nothing more than a lab error. It was simply one of those inconveniences that couldn't be avoided, so I obediently returned to the Kaiser Permanente Breast Center for a second mammogram. After this second film was developed, a stony-faced technician led me down the hall to the radiologist's office.

The radiologist had both of my mammograms fastened to a lighted panel on the wall. He pointed to the questionable area on the film. It certainly did appear vague. In fact, to me, it didn't look like anything at all. The doctor explained that this mass was probably nothing, but to be on the safe side, I should have a biopsy. Of the two choices offered, I selected the needle biopsy. Painless. I'd be in and out in the time it would take to have my hair done.

He then asked me if I had a surgeon. Why in the world would I have a surgeon? I blindly selected Dr. Janice Schilling mostly because I liked the pleasant sound of her name. The radiologist said I had made a wise choice. The biopsy was scheduled for the following Tuesday morning.

I had a stereotactic needle biopsy that entailed removing nine core samples of tissue from my breast. They had lied about it being painless, but once the procedure was over I needed only a few Tylenol tablets to manage the discomfort. Dr. Schilling called two days later.

"Mrs. Rosen," she said, "I'm afraid I have bad news."

"Cancer?" I whispered. My own voice sounded like a distant echo trembling through my head. It wasn't my voice at all.

"Yes, I'm afraid so."

I sat in stupefied silence while her words registered in my brain. Breast cancer? I had breast cancer? How could this be possible? I was suddenly a skydiver who'd hit the ground without a parachute.

I finally said, "What happens next?"

"How soon can you get to my office?" she asked.

"Thirty minutes."

"I'll be waiting for you."

I went to find my husband, Morrie. He was sitting at the kitchen table reading the newspaper, having a cup of coffee. When I told him, the color drained from his face as if the news had somehow bleached the life out of him. He took me in his arms and held me. I felt numb, too numb even to cry. We got into the car and drove the twenty miles to the hospital, mostly in silence.

As promised, Dr. Schilling was waiting in her office. She came from behind her massive desk, effectively removing any physical barriers, and sat next to me. She frequently reached out and touched me. The radiologist had been right. I'd made a very wise choice when I'd selected this gentle woman to lead me through the alien territory of breast cancer.

Dr. Schilling explained my pathology report, informing me that I had a cancerous tumor in one of the many lobules (milk glands) in my right breast. The cancer was described as invasive or infiltrating, which meant it had spread out of the lobule where it had started, growing into the surrounding tissue. Surgery was my best option. Dr. Schilling was optimistic; however, because the cancer had been discovered early. She went on to clarify the pros and cons of lumpectomy versus mastectomy.

My world had just fallen apart, and yet I was supposed to make calm, rational decisions and select my preferred form of surgery. I sat there feeling strangely detached from reality. I was hearing unfamiliar terms like infiltrating lobular carcinoma, estrogen receptor stains, lymph nodes, radiation, and chemotherapy, but my mind was still wrestling with that one word: cancer.

Not so long ago, cancer was a word that wasn't spoken. When it happened to others, we discussed the patient's prognosis in hushed whispers, without ever really uttering the word. Cancer was just too dreadful, too frightening. This couldn't be happening to me, yet there I was sitting in a surgeon's office, hearing that word over and over.

I scheduled surgery for the following Monday morning, December 4, 1995. Next, I was given instructions to go through the maze of procedures called pre-op. Following the blood work, X-rays, and an EKG, I met with a nurse who explained what was going to happen to me before, during, and after surgery. I was given written instructions in case I forgot anything. I held onto those instructions for dear life because I'd forgotten every word she'd said even before we left her office.

Half way through my pre-op appointments, we went to the hospital cafeteria for a bite to eat. I forced myself to swallow without tasting the food. I was functioning like a robot. By the time we finally exited the hospital, it had grown late and a deep purple haze blurred the western sky. Like the evening sky, everything in my line of vision had become a blur. Morrie had his arm around my shoulder as we slowly trudged through the near-empty parking lot. We barely spoke and when we did, it was in a whisper.

That night I looked in the mirror and the full impact of this very long day finally registered. I had cancer. I wondered whether I would die. I wasn't ready to die. I was only fifty-four.

Two years earlier we'd moved from Los Angeles to Thousand Oaks, California, seeking a smaller, less hectic community away from the bustle of the city, and Morrie had retired from his job as a stockbroker. Our life since the move had bordered on perfection, and we certainly had not planned on having something as insidious as cancer invading our idyllic new lifestyle. An old Jewish saying kept popping into my mind: "You want to make God laugh? Tell him your plans."

I had two grown children, Scott and Nancy, a stepdaughter, Deborah, and four beautiful granddaughters. I wanted to see my grandchildren grow up. I wanted to dance at their weddings. Suddenly, my family became the most important thing in my life.

My son, Scott Rosen, has always been a tremendous source of joy and pride. He developed a marvelous sense of humor as a child, and as an adult his wit and wry humor keep me smiling. Dedicated and completely earnest about his academic studies, Scott has earned two masters degrees and now works as a reference librarian and assistant professor at Azusa Pacific University. His generous assistance and support with my writing career have been an undeniable blessing.

My daughter, Nancy De Channes, is a delightful natural reflection of me. Through Nancy, I have enjoyed seeing myself as a child, a teenager, and now a young mother all over again. She is so passionate about everything she does that, as a child, her gentle heart cast her into the role of neighborhood Earth Mother, adopting stray cats, dogs, and people. Like her brother, Nancy is sensitive, conscientious, and considerate.

I consider my stepdaughter, Deborah Kiel, an extraordinary gift. When I married Morrie she came into my life as a bonus, albeit a teenage one. Since then I have watched her grow into a lovely, self-assured woman who has become a precious friend as well as my daughter.

I had taught English on the junior and senior high school level for a number of years and then went on to become a writer. It had never occurred to me that someday I might write about cancer. I now understood that whatever I had planned for the immediate future had to be placed on "hold." I realized that some of the many things I wanted to accomplish in life might never come to pass.

The day of surgery I was first taken into radiology and a localized wire probe was inserted into my breast with the aid of mammography equipment. This instrument was supposed to guide Dr. Schilling to the exact location of my tumor. With a long wire protruding from my breast like some bionic creature from a sci-fi movie, I was prepped for surgery and anesthesia was initiated. I remember being wheeled into the operating room before everything went blank.

Dr. Schilling performed a lumpectomy and removed seventeen lymph nodes from under my right arm. Lymph nodes, chains of little glands that cluster together like a bunch of grapes, carry lymphatic fluid throughout the body as part of the immune system. If cancer cells escape into the lymph nodes, the fluid can transport the cancer and deposit it in other parts of the body.

I spent some time in the recovery room, and then, after I began to display signs of slight coherence, I was released to go home. Home sounded good at the time, but once the anesthesia had completely worn off, I began to feel extreme pain in my armpit and down my right arm. No amount of pain pills or bags of frozen peas tucked under my arm gave me any relief.

Morrie called Dr. Schilling. She explained that the Jackson-Pratt drain (JP drain to those who understand the lingo) that had been inserted into the site of my incision to drain off any fluid build-up was possibly pressing against a nerve. Loud and clear, that drain was pressing against something. That night I hoped I wouldn't overdose on all the painkillers I was swallowing.

But the pain medication did not take effect, and my pain simply would not go away. Dr. Schilling had ordered a stronger medication, but the pain had become so unbearable that I cried whenever Morrie helped me out of bed to use the bathroom. This went on for three days until our son Scott decided that I must see my surgeon at once, rather than wait for my upcoming scheduled appointment. His wife Ellen stayed home with their infant daughter Natalie while Scott took charge and drove Morrie and me back to Kaiser for an emergency visit.

Dr. Schilling agreed with Scott, and she removed the JP drain three days early. That was the good news. She'd also received my pathology report, and it was the bad news. My lymph nodes showed no evidence of cancer, but all the supposedly healthy margins of tissue surrounding the tumor had contained cancer cells. We scheduled a bigger and better lumpectomy for Monday December 18.

Round Two

Exactly two weeks after the first lumpectomy, I returned to the same operating room. The same friends showed up at the hospital and kept vigil with Morrie and our daughter Nancy. My friend Mary Johnson must have read and corrected two hundred student essays while I was in surgery. Ruth Baker and Betty Rabin Fung were also there, along with Morrie's old army buddy, Jules Posner and his wife, Leatrice.

This time I went home without a drain and once again resumed the process of getting well. After my incision healed, I would begin radiation treatments. The first few days went well, and I was blessed with a virtual shower of cards and flowers. Ruth Baker called me every single day, and she organized many of my teacher friends into my own personal "Meals on Wheels" service. Dozens of friends prepared and delivered a wonderful assortment of home-cooked foods. Then the second pathology report arrived in Dr. Schilling's office.

The only definite thing you can say about cancer is that it isn't fair. The one-inch margins of tissue that had been removed from around the original surgery site all showed signs of atypical lobular carcinoma. More cancer. We had to go back and try again.

We met with Dr. Schilling, and although she said she was willing to make another attempt to save my breast with an even larger excision around the original lumpectomy, I decided to have the entire breast removed. Breasts are nice, but I wasn't ready to die for one.

I also met with an oncologist, Dr. Edward Chang. Much like Dr. Schilling, Dr. Chang is a wonderfully calm, soft-spoken physician who cares a great deal about his patients. He did a thorough physical exam and talked about my coming mastectomy. He explained that I wouldn't need radiation if the entire breast was removed, but I would have to take a drug called Tamoxifen, an oral chemotherapy that inhibits the growth of estrogen-sensitive breast cancer cells. The lab had already determined that my cancer was estrogen-sensitive, so Tamoxifen would be my constant companion for the next five years. At least Dr. Chang was figuring my life expectancy in terms of <u>years</u> (rather than months), and that was a slight degree of comfort.

While Dr. Chang did his best to alleviate my fears, I slipped into the vast Bermuda Triangle of my mind. How had a disease as loathsome as cancer moved into my breast in the first place? Had I been exposed to something that caused cancer to grow in my body, or was it just a stroke of rotten luck? Had microscopic cancer cells already spread to parts unknown? Was it in my brain or lungs? Would it attack my other breast?

I knew that many people survived cancer. Dr. Chang said that about forty percent of all cancer patients are still alive five years after diagnosis, and with early detection my chances were probably even better. But how could I be certain I would be one of the lucky ones? I had so many questions for which there didn't seem to be any answers.

My third surgery within thirty days had been scheduled for January 4, 1996. I had to go home and wait, wondering how I would survive the next few days. At one moment I was openly angry. Then suddenly my emotional roller coaster would dip way down to a sensation of complete helplessness. Feeling powerless was usually accompanied by an overwhelming sense of impending loss. Why did it have to be so hard?

The night before surgery, Morrie kissed my breast and said goodbye to it. Sounds silly now, I guess, but it was the most loving, tender thing he could have done. He wasn't upset about my losing the breast if it meant he would still have his wife. I'd heard about men who were unable to stay with a mate who'd lost a breast and therefore part of her femininity to cancer. I imagine a woman whose husband flees to lessen his own pain must feel a lot like a soldier who receives a "Dear John" letter in the midst of enemy fire. I was grateful Morrie could see beyond the superficial.

"Everything will be all right," Morrie said.

I whispered, "I know," and then moments later I fell apart.

I cried myself to sleep knowing I would spend the following night in the hospital. I had graduated from an outpatient to an in-patient. I had arrived. I had the word CANCER stamped in red letters on the cover of my medical chart. The chart itself had grown considerably in thickness. I just wanted my cancer days to be over.

Dr. Schilling removed my right breast. A modified mastectomy involves excising the breast, the lining over the chest muscles, and sometimes the minor pectoral muscle. My lymph nodes had already been removed during the first surgery or they would have been included.

The pathologist discovered microscopic cancer in every quadrant of the breast, so it turned out my having the mastectomy had been the correct decision. Although the less radical lumpectomy seems to be the preferred method of eliminating breast cancer nowadays, it was clearly not the right choice for me. Unfortunately, this can't be determined in advance in most cases because microscopic disease is not detectable until the tissue is examined under a microscope.

As the days following surgery progressed, I found myself surrounded by family and caring friends. My friend Pat Klein who'd had a mastectomy some twenty years earlier traveled over 400 miles from Palo Alto, California, to be with me and to offer her support. I'd never felt so loved.

Ruth Baker, who teaches math but specializes in wonderful matzo ball soup, came over and cooked up her specialty. Betty Rabin Fung, a home economics teacher, delivered a sensational low-fat dinner, which included something from every one of the basic 4 food groups. I'd always been able to count on my long-time friends Betty and Ruth, and they continued to be there for me with meals and their unwavering friendship.

Friends came from all over Southern California to cheer me up, and I received dozens of cards every day. One especially touching note came from Susan Stephenson, a member of Sisters in Crime and fellow mystery writer. She wrote in part, ".... Though lonely you may feel, you are not—and never will be—alone. All of us with breasts and the intelligence to understand our vulnerability are quietly at your side."

Maya Ashworth came from northern California, and Marylou Mahar flew down from Oregon. The phone never stopped ringing. It didn't take long to learn who my real friends were, and I felt blessed to feel so much love.

In the midst of all this attention, however, I soon realized I was burning up with fever. My chest wall had become infected, and the skin adjacent to the incision felt hot to the touch. Dr. Schilling prescribed oral antibiotics, but the pain just kept getting worse. After a week, my fever spiked even higher. Dr. Schilling again asked how quickly we could get to the hospital.

We arrived at Dr. Schilling's office within the Kaiser Medical Facility while she was in the middle of her lunch. Her sandwich set aside, she immediately examined me and explained that I would have to be placed on high dosage intravenous antibiotics for at least eight days.

"But I don't want to be in the hospital for eight days," I said.

"Unless you have someone at home who can administer antibiotics through an IV, you have no choice," Dr. Schilling said.

"My husband can do that," I blurted out.

Morrie knew a lot about many different things, but running an IV wasn't one of them. In spite of this, he volunteered to be trained for home infusion, a process that took several hours. An infusion nurse inserted an IV port that Morrie would use into the back of my left hand. She then taught him how to administer the antibiotics via the port, a procedure he would follow around the clock. Now I was praying for Morrie to have the strength to get us through the next eight days.

Morrie carried a whole crate of sterile tubing, clamps, needle syringes, alcohol wipes, and plastic bags filled with powerful antibiotics to our car. We went straight home and unloaded the crate. Within moments, our bathroom looked as if it had been converted into a Red Cross center. I soon learned that Morrie took the "in sickness and in health" part of our marriage vows quite seriously.

He used a syringe of saline solution to flush the port before he carefully connected a plastic tube to the back of my hand. He took extreme caution, making certain there were no air bubbles in the tubing. We both held our breath as he released the clamp to begin the drip. It worked! And thus began eight days from Hell.

Being tethered by tubes to bag after bag of antibiotics was sheer misery. By the end of the week I was feeling very sorry for myself, but the infection did finally disappear. Maybe now the worst was over, but it was hard to feel optimistic in light of all that had happened to me. I realized that I was recovering physically, but I also knew my emotional recovery would not be quite so easy.

I wondered whether it was now okay for me to get back to the life I'd put on hold during the last six weeks, or was I missing the point? Perhaps that old life of mine no longer existed. Perhaps cancer is more than a terrible disease. Could it be a catalyst that causes people who survive it to reevaluate and restructure their lives? I did a lot of reading and a lot of thinking. I gradually came to a point where I stopped feeling miserable because I had cancer and focused instead on how lucky I was that my cancer had been detected early.

I spent time each day doing some guided imagery as described by Dr. O. Carl Simonton in his book, <u>Getting Well Again</u>. I visualized myself in a beautiful outdoor refuge filled with an abundance of flowers. This image usually filtered down to resemble our own flower garden that Morrie and I had so carefully nurtured. Once I was in this peaceful, floral haven, I would picture myself well and completely free of disease.

My friend Linda Ruhle helped me master this process, and even after she'd moved from Los Angeles to a little town named Ten Sleep, Wyoming, she continued to guide me long distance. Linda had cured herself of viral encephalomyelitis (an inflammation of the brain and spinal cord which is an incurable disease according to the medical community) and has since used her mind-over-body knowledge to heal others. Together we explored the mind-body connection with the understanding that a positive state of mind could lead to wellness. She taught me to believe that my thinking could affect something as small as a single cell in my body.

I read everything about cancer I could get my hands on including <u>Dr. Susan Love's Breast Book</u> by Susan M. Love, M.D. I learned more about breast cancer than I ever wanted to know, but I also discovered there is far too much about all cancers that remains unknown. Despite all the advances in cancer research in recent years, medical science does not always know what causes a healthy cell to become cancerous. Although researchers seem to be getting closer to a cure with each passing year, especially in areas such as gene therapy and immunotherapy, we still haven't cracked the code of cancer.

I, for one, thought I had done everything right. I ate broccoli. I avoided red meat. I didn't work around pesticides or other chemicals. I didn't even smoke. I rarely drank alcohol. Breast cancer didn't run in my family. It became clear to me that cancer has multiple causes and multiple risk factors. My cancer obviously had something to do with my genetic makeup, environmental factors, and the state of my immune system. Perhaps my emotions and life experiences also colored the picture to a degree. I didn't find answers to all of my questions, but I did finally decide that at least I could rest easy knowing that whatever had caused my breast cancer was not my fault.

About two months went by. I set only short-term goals for myself, so I could see at least a tiny bit of progress in the routine things I tried to accomplish each day. I began attending a weekly support group for breast cancer patients and survivors and got to know some women who were handling their disease quite easily and others who dissolved into tears at every meeting.

I listened to their stories, relating to their fears, caring for them as individuals. We exchanged phone numbers and called one another whenever we felt a need to connect with someone who really understood the whole gamut of crazy feelings and fear that accompany breast cancer. We had all learned that as much as family and friends tried to be supportive, they couldn't understand what we were going through no matter how hard they tried. Expecting others to understand wouldn't even be fair, and since cancer couldn't be the only topic of conversation with friends, we needed the safety of the support group where we could open up and express our fears. The help I received from the other cancer patients was something unique that I was certain I couldn't find elsewhere.

I finally felt as if I were healing emotionally as well as physically. I gradually resumed many of my former activities. I had lost most of the feeling under my right arm, but I had no trouble using the arm. I joined the YMCA and attended their water fitness exercise classes. Morrie and I took long walks. I was enjoying each day, feeling that life was once again pretty good.

I returned to my writing, picking up the pieces of a novel I'd started before I was diagnosed. I also began to write about my feelings regarding the cancer, sketchy notes that made little sense at the time, but later found their way into this book. Even if these words were never published, I believed that a cleansing of sorts came from forging my innermost thoughts into words. Sentences are usually pretty standard. Subject—verb—object. Sentences are tidy little groups of words. Reducing cancer into sentences, a form that I could understand and control, removed some of its menacing power over my life.

Three months had gone by since my mastectomy. Then one morning I discovered a hard lump in my abdomen.

Rosemary's Baby

It was a Saturday. Morrie was an early riser and was probably downstairs reading the paper. I'd gotten up and gone to the bathroom, but I then crawled back into our cozy bed and decided that another half-hour of sleep wouldn't be a bad idea. Sleep didn't come instantly, so I eventually rolled over onto my back.

A mocking bird called.

A dog barked.

The breast cancer had taught me not to put pressures on myself, so I'd had no problem just lying there, gazing through the partially opened vertical blinds. On a distant hill the branches of tall pines flickered in the wind against the overcast steel-gray morning sky. I wondered if the clouds would eventually give way to rain.

I don't know why my hand drifted onto my lower abdomen. Maybe I had felt a slight pressure? Perhaps my hand had been guided to the spot by an unseen force? I don't know what prompted me to explore, but I gently pushed my fingertips into the area just above the pubic bone and slightly to my left, and there it was. A hard lump the size of a walnut.

I'd read that breast cancer was frequently accompanied by colon cancer. In fact Sandy Grofsky, a woman in the breast cancer support group, had been diagnosed with colon cancer only one month earlier. I felt for the lump again. It was still there.

My bladder was empty. My stomach was empty. It had to be my colon, I reasoned, without taking the time to envision a diagram of the body's digestive system. I concluded that the lump was probably nothing more than a knot of hard stool lodged somewhere in the intestine. It was Saturday; I couldn't reach Dr. Chang. I would check the lump again Sunday morning.

I spent the day out of kilter, my brain feeling somehow disconnected from the rest of me, but I went through the motions of household chores to get my mind off the mysterious new lump. When I awakened Sunday morning, I checked the same spot. My bowels had moved, but the lump hadn't. I definitely wasn't feeling hard stool in the intestine.

I finally asked Morrie to check the lump. Maybe my imagination was running rampant. I couldn't possibly have another cancerous tumor just three months after the tumor in my breast, could I? Morrie barely touched the spot with two fingertips, but he felt it, too.

I didn't know what I'd found, but I knew it could not be ignored. Ignoring this lump or even taking my time about having it checked by a doctor simply was not one of my options.

Monday morning I telephoned Dr. Chang's office. I made an appointment for Wednesday and continued to spend most of my time worrying about the lump. I kept telling myself that Dr. Chang would reassure me. He would proclaim this lump was the friendliest lump in town. We'd have a good laugh when he identified it as . . . what? All logic and reasoning skills had flown right out of my head.

Dr. Chang examined me. He wasn't laughing at all. "I didn't feel this lump last month," he said.

My eyes filled with tears.

"It must be a cyst, but it's probably nothing to worry about."

"Could it be the breast cancer?" I asked.

"No, it's not the breast cancer, and I doubt it's any kind of cancer, but I want to order an ultrasound, just to be sure."

My legs took me downstairs in the medical center to the department where ultrasound tests are scheduled. A few days later, a radiologist administered the ultrasound. He said Dr. Chang would discuss the results with me, but he did admit the lump was in my left ovary. He also said I shouldn't worry. He assured me that eighty percent of all ovarian cysts are not malignant. Dr. Chang wanted confirmation from a gynecologist, so that appointment was arranged. The gynecologist examined me and studied the film from the ultrasound.

"Can you tell what it is?" I asked.

She looked me squarely in the eye. "What I see on the ultrasound is not consistent with a benign cyst."

This woman apparently believed in bringing out the big guns right from the start. I didn't cry. The way I was feeling went much deeper than tears. I said, "Then you're saying it looks like cancer?"

"Of course we can't be absolutely certain until the lab puts it under a microscope, but yes, it looks like cancer."

"Putting it under a microscope means more surgery."

She nodded. "Dr. Chang will put you in touch with a surgeon, one who specializes in gynecological oncology."

Feeling like Dorothy venturing toward OZ, I was off to see yet another physician. We drove about fifty miles to the Kaiser facility near Hollywood where I was assigned to a highly skilled gynecological surgeon, Dr. Neal Semrad. Dr. Semrad was always followed by a procession of young interns or resident doctors who were training under him, and his entourage squeezed into the tiny examination room and formed a circle around me.

Dr. Semrad referred to my ultrasound and explained my case to the other doctors. He continued his lecture as he carefully probed my abdomen and performed a pelvic exam. Next, he instructed one of the interns to examine me also. When he'd finished, the younger man nodded gravely. I guess I was the highlight of the day for this medical team, and I suddenly understood how the sideshow "freaks" in traveling carnivals must feel as curiosity-seekers gape at them.

Dr. Semrad ordered a CT scan, and it was arranged for the following Sunday morning. Surgery was scheduled for the day after the scan, Monday April 29, 1996.

Waiting those few days for the surgery was nerve-wracking to say the least. I remember at one point I looked in the mirror and thought to myself, Lord help me, but if this is as bad as I think it is, I'm going to die. My heart felt heavy. I wasn't ready for my life to be over.

I'd never really thought about my own death before. Somehow death was a distant possibility that wouldn't require any serious thought on my part for many years to come. I'd certainly never thought that I'd die from cancer. Cancer simply never entered my mind. Cancer happened to other people. If anything, my concerns should have been over the heart disease that seemed to run rampant on my father's side of the family.

Anxiety was eating away at me. I wondered if my insides were actually as hollow as they felt. Was this the way the average nervous breakdown began? I thought I couldn't live through another day with this threat hanging over me, but I soon discovered that I survived not only that particular day, but the next one as well.

For the rest of the week, I got up in the morning, brushed my teeth, ate breakfast, and followed my usual routine. I learned that somehow life goes on. I even went to the breast cancer support group to discuss my new fears. By now we'd become friends who'd joined together to fight the common enemy: cancer. I surprised myself by living through each day, knowing that I was facing yet another major surgery and perhaps more cancer.

Through all of this, Morrie did a fairly good job of trying to maintain a happy-go-lucky façade. His smile was so constant you would've thought he was the Grand Marshall of the Rose Parade. Of course, he didn't fool me for a moment. Morrie was heartsick about the prospect of my having another cancer, but the word didn't cross his lips very often. We were both reeling while desperately trying to assure one another that everything was fine and dandy. Morrie carried on as usual as if nothing were wrong, but I knew he was miserable.

Naturally, I'd continued checking the lump on a daily basis, and in less than three weeks it had grown so rapidly that I was actually able to feel the changes in its size from day to day. I don't know why tumors are always compared to pieces of fruit, but my walnut had grown into a good-sized plum, then days later it had taken on the proportions of an apple. The day I went into the hospital for surgery, it was as big as a large grapefruit. How could anything grow that rapidly? I jokingly referred to the monster I was carrying in my abdomen as Rosemary's Baby.

Joking aside, the threat of imminent death had released a torrent of inner strength I never knew I had. Although no one had told me in so many words, I somehow became aware that fighting back would be a critical part of my recovery. I came into the world kicking and screaming, and it now made sense that I should continue on that same course.

I tried to channel positive energy from my mind right down to the core of Rosemary's Baby. I remembered that positive thinking could affect something as small as a single cell. Positive thinking could make me well. I also tried to funnel a brilliant white light, which I imagined emanating from somewhere on high, down into my body. I was spending a lot of time either preoccupied with healing mental exercises or prayer. Positive thinking and prayer seemed to go naturally hand in hand.

My friends kept telling me not to worry. Everyone said that ovarian cysts are usually benign. As I was being prepped for surgery, the nurse even assured me that my cyst was probably not cancerous. She said they remove benign cysts every day.

My mind was growing fuzzy from the sedative she'd injected into my IV to relax me, but the words of the consulting gynecologist I'd seen the previous week continued to haunt me. What she'd seen on the ultrasound was not consistent with a benign cyst. It didn't matter that it would be highly unusual for me to have another primary cancer so soon after the breast cancer. By now, no matter what anyone said, I knew that I had ovarian cancer.

I went into surgery repeating a mantra in my mind. Over and over I told myself: "I have cancer, but I'm going to beat it. I have cancer, but I'm going to survive."

University of Cancer

When I finally awakened from the anesthesia, I was vaguely aware of faces surrounding my hospital bed. Morrie was there, of course, and our daughter Nancy. Nancy dabbed a cool, damp cloth against my parched lips. A nurse adjusted a stream of medication that was flowing through an IV tube into my arm. My eyes swam in and out of focus until I recognized that my stepdaughter Deborah Kiel and our good friends Ruth and Allen Baker and Betty Rabin Fung were also in the room. I was in pain, and I was terribly thirsty, but my discomfort could wait. Good or bad news, I wanted to know about the cancer.

When Morrie noticed that I had opened my eyes, he leaned over and kissed me on the forehead. It seemed to take every bit of strength I could muster just to form a few words.

I finally said, "Was it cancer?"

"Yes," he said.

With that fact established, a strange sensation washed over me. Perhaps I was simply stoned from the anesthesia, but there was no real terror or even the sense of bewilderment that I'd felt when I first heard the diagnosis of breast cancer. It was as if I'd resigned myself to yet another disease, simply another battle that had to be won. My having this new cancer wasn't fair, but then I'd already established the fact that cancer, like life itself, does not go out of its way to be fair. At the same time, a sixth sense also told me that I must stop thinking the worst.

I'd made up my mind I was going to survive, so positive thinking had to remain a major part of my treatment. While in the hospital when I could do nothing more than stare at the ceiling, I spent the hours repeating my mantra. It wasn't simply my wishing away the cancer. By believing that I could get well as Linda Ruhle had taught me, I was making a mind-body connection that I believed could strengthen my immune system enough to fight off any remaining cancer cells.

In spite of my inner shift in thinking, I knew I still had a long way to recovery. The abdominal surgery that involved a hysterectomy as well as removing the tumor, both ovaries and both fallopian tubes was so much more painful than the breast surgery, and getting in and out of bed alone was an almost impossible feat. Dr. Semrad came to see me and explained that he was feeling extremely encouraged about the tumor he'd removed from my abdomen.

"It was very close to the point when it would most likely rupture," he said, "but I think we got it out in time. The external capsule appeared intact, but we'll know more when I get the pathology report."

Dr. Semrad was smiling when he left my room, so I had even more reason to feel hopeful. This time I spent five days in the hospital and went home with my stomach held together by a painful row of nasty looking wire staples. Morrie helped me up the stairs to our bedroom, and I didn't step foot downstairs for a week. Again our friends delivered wonderful home-cooked meals to our home, and Morrie or Nancy carried trays upstairs to serve me in bed.

Everything in my life had changed. I'd been ripped from a fairly pleasant routine of daily activities back into a sickroom. Again my writing, our long walks, playing with the grandchildren, everything I enjoyed had to be placed on hold.

During this time it was easy to fall into the pattern of asking myself "Why me?" Although I kept telling myself that God doesn't hand out cancer on a first-come first-served basis, I couldn't imagine what had been responsible for bringing on both breast and ovarian cancers. I knew a high-fat diet plays a part in cancer, but I'd been fairly sensible about my diet for years. Perhaps it's necessary to start thinking low fat when you're a child in order to guarantee that your diet won't be the cause of cancer.

From what I'd read, there were no clear-cut definitive causes of most cancers except for skin cancer, which results from too much exposure to the sun, and of course the many different forms of cancer that are directly attributed to tobacco.

Thirty percent of all cancers are supposed to be caused by tobacco, and, in light of what we know about tobacco and cancer, I can't understand why anyone would smoke. Recently I spotted a sign along the freeway that stated: "500,000,000 People Alive Today Will Die From Tobacco." That's half a billion people!

Tobacco-related cancer is the leading cause of death in the United States that could be prevented with self-discipline. The fact remains, however, that an individual has to have a strong resolution in order to kick the addiction. (The individual also has to believe that cancer could actually strike him or her personally. Regarding cancer, many people live in complete denial.)

Nevertheless, in spite of the millions who will die from tobacco-related cancers, I couldn't blame my own cancer on tobacco because I'd never smoked, and I even made a point of avoiding second-hand smoke.

As far as breast and ovarian cancers are concerned, genetic factors cause many women to inherit the disease, but researchers claim that heredity accounts for no more than seven to ten percent of all cases. My mother had died of leukemia, but no one in my family had ever suffered from breast or ovarian cancer. Both of my cancers were classified as "sporadic," which is usually the case with most cancers. In fact with breast cancer, the literature I'd read used the term "increased risk" rather than "cause" in relation to things like excessive alcohol consumption, fat in the diet, and exposure to radiation.

Women in Holland, for example, reportedly have an elevated rate of breast cancer. Researchers attribute this tendency partially to the high consumption of dairy products in their country. Breast cancer is also linked to hormone replacement (estrogen replacement therapy or ERT), and unfortunately, for the last year I had taken estrogen pills to reduce the side effects of my approaching menopause.

The increased risk factors for ovarian cancer, like breast cancer, include consumption of high-fat foods, again especially dairy products. With ovarian cancer, not having children or having them late in life, never having used oral contraceptives, or never breast feeding also seem to increase a woman's risk. (Oral contraceptives, like pregnancy and breast-feeding, inhibit ovulation.) None of these factors applied to me.

The use of talc, as in talcum powder, also could be involved in the development of ovarian cancer. The tiny particles of talc found in dusting powders are much like asbestos, and these fibers can travel up the fallopian tubes to the ovaries the same way asbestos particles creep into the lungs, causing lung cancer. I thought back to all the internal pelvic exams I'd had while pregnant and remembered how they used to pack surgical latex gloves in talc. Doctors claim that the risk of using talc is actually quite insignificant, but I've also noticed that pharmaceutical supply companies no longer package surgical gloves in this manner.

I reconciled myself to the fact that despite doing all the "right" things, a person can still get cancer. I wasn't overweight and I didn't drink more than one or two glasses of wine per month, but I'd had my share of potato chips and ice cream in my life. I probably would never know for certain why I contracted two cancers, one right after the other. I'd heard about a woman who'd been diagnosed with breast and ovarian cancer, both on the very same day, so I learned not to complain. No matter how bad a situation seems, things could always be worse.

At night, when my abdominal pain seemed to intensify, Morrie was reluctant to sleep in our bed with me, fearing his tossing and turning might cause me even more pain. He refused to sleep in our guestroom—claiming it was too far away from me—when it was actually just thirty feet down the hall. He solved the problem by unrolling our portable futon and sleeping on the floor next to me. When Morrie wasn't performing one of his nursing duties, he was right there by my side.

My usual attempts to maintain an orderly home faded to an almost casual curiosity about whether the kitchen would require sandblasting when I returned to it. Gradually I came to realize that a lot more than our sleeping arrangements had changed. I finally decided that I really didn't care whether the kitchen was a mess. I could handle only one disaster at a time, and at that moment I was concentrating on surviving cancer. Things I normally would have worried about no longer mattered.

When I finally returned to the kitchen for my first meal downstairs, I found things were out of place but in a tidy sort of way. I didn't care. No sandblasting was required, and I finally realized there are many things in life that are more important than orderly kitchens. My priorities had shifted, and I was now kinder to myself and I hoped gentler with others.

After another week of recovery, Morrie and I traveled back to Dr. Semrad's office for a follow-up consultation. Nancy and Scott went along. First, a doctor removed the staples from my abdomen. At that point I learned that when a doctor says you're going to feel a tiny pinch, translate that to mean momentary-but-savage agony. After the staples had been removed, I got dressed and the four of us were ushered into a small conference room.

We talked with Dr. Semrad and one of his assistants for over an hour. Scott had apparently done some research of his own, and he posed many pertinent questions that I hadn't thought to ask. Nancy was also armed with a list of essential questions. Scott and Nancy were determined to understand what we as a family were facing.

Dr. Semrad explained the pathology report in great detail. I'd learned that only twenty percent of all ovarian cancers are diagnosed in stage I (stage IV being worst). Another ten percent are diagnosed at stage II, which included me. Most cases, however, are not discovered until the tumor has burst, propelling the cancer all over the abdominal cavity.

But even when the outer covering of the tumor appears to be intact, it's possible for fast growing cancer cells to escape the capsule and travel elsewhere. For this reason, Dr. Semrad had performed an abdominal wash while I was in surgery. During this procedure a sterile saline solution was injected throughout my abdominal cavity. Cells that might be impossible to detect otherwise can be "washed out" in this manner. This fluid was then recovered from my abdominal cavity and examined by the pathologist.

I had bizarre visions of the surgeon hosing down a patio or a sidewalk, but I was assured that this procedure was a very important one and my results in particular were remarkable. Not only had my tumor been removed supposedly intact but the wash was free of cancer cells. Dr. Semrad had also performed biopsies on other organs as well as the underside of my diaphragm. In addition to excising my uterus, ovaries, and fallopian tubes, Dr. Semrad had removed my appendix, pelvic lymph nodes, and omentum. (The omentum is fatty tissue connected to the upper colon and it frequently will capture free-floating tumor cells.)

This meticulous surgical staging had discovered no additional cancer cells in my abdominal cavity. Wow! We had reason for celebrating, and I was thrilled . . . but not for long.

Dr. Semrad said, yes, my news was good, except for one tiny glitch. My particular ovarian cancer that had grown so rapidly was a very rare form of the disease called a clear cell carcinoma. Clear cell, even when it is still confined to the ovary, tends to be the most challenging of the various types of ovarian cancer in terms of treatment and long-term survival for the patient.

Because this cancer is so rare, statistical information on clear cell is almost non-existent, and the necessary treatment to prevent a recurrence seems to involve a lot of guesswork. As a result, Dr. Semrad recommended an extensive program of chemotherapy for me.

I'd had no idea that there were thirty different kinds of ovarian cancer in the first place. And who would've suspected that I'd be blessed with a rare form of it? There was so much about this disease that I didn't understand, but I had just enrolled in the University of Cancer and I had a feeling I was soon going to learn.

The Silent Killer

I had learned what little I knew about ovarian cancer from reading Gilda Radner's autobiography, It's Always Something. Like most fans of "Saturday Night Live," I'd been stunned when I'd learned that the popular comedienne had ovarian cancer, then shocked when she later died from the disease on May 20, 1989. With her unfortunate death, however, ovarian cancer was finally drawn out of the shadows and openly discussed in magazine and newspaper articles.

In her book, Gilda Radner described round after round of medical appointments as a result of her experiencing many of the symptoms of ovarian cancer. For over a year, she was treated for Epstein-Barr virus, a disease she didn't have, while the real culprit, ovarian cancer, grew out of control.

Sadly, even today, most cases of ovarian cancer are misdiagnosed as something non-cancerous like irritable bowel syndrome or gastritis. Because of this, ovarian cancer is often called the Silent Killer. According to the American Cancer Society and the Ovarian Cancer National Alliance, in the United States ovarian cancer strikes one out of every 55 women or 1.8 percent of the female population as compared to the more widespread breast cancer that attacks one out of every eight.

Ovarian cancer has symptoms, but they are usually just vague enough that the disease is not properly diagnosed until it has spread to other organs, leaving the woman with a very slim chance of survival. In fact, 60 percent of all women with ovarian cancer have stage III disease, which has already spread to the abdomen when they are first diagnosed, and another 10 percent will have stage IV, spread to the liver or somewhere else beyond the abdomen. (I have since learned that over seventy-five percent of all malpractice law suits deal with delayed cancer diagnosis.)

Some of the most common symptoms of ovarian cancer include intestinal gas, backaches, bloating, and a general feeling of exhaustion. I don't think there's a woman alive who hasn't felt all of the above symptoms at one time or another. Some women are guaranteed these annoyances every month during their years of menstruation. It would certainly be normal for a woman to put off seeing a doctor for many months if the above complaints were the only symptoms she had, and unfortunately that's exactly what happens. As benign as these symptoms may appear, they should never be ignored.

Other symptoms of ovarian cancer include nausea, indigestion, constipation, or diarrhea. Some women report frequent or urgent urination or menstrual disorders. Pain, especially during intercourse, is often the last problem to appear, but many women report no pain at all.

Then there's the symptom that alerted me, actually discovering the tumor myself. Medical researchers claim that by the time a tumor can be felt, it has already lived seventy-five percent of its ultimate life. I was told that it is almost unheard of for ovarian cancer to be accidentally discovered by the patient the way mine was detected. Women simply don't bother to probe their abdomens in search of lumps the way they do self-exams on their breasts. Perhaps they should.

The symptoms of ovarian cancer are subtle, persistent, and usually increase if left unattended. The Ovarian Cancer National Alliance advocates that any time one of these symptoms continues for more than two or three weeks, a woman should seek medical attention, insisting upon a pelvic exam, a CA 125 tumor marker blood test, and a transvaginal sonogram or ultrasound. It's my belief that if a woman feels something is wrong with her body, it probably is. Women need to be aware that ovarian cancer is called The Silent Killer for a very good reason, and we must listen when it whispers.

I may have gotten away with just the surgery (clinically referred to as debulking) if I'd had a less mysterious form of ovarian cancer. The prospect of chemotherapy was frightening, but I was still feeling positive. Not knowing much about chemotherapy, I decided I needed to do a little research.

According to M. Steven Piver, M.D. in his book Gilda's Disease, written with Gene Wilder, chemotherapy was first discovered by accident during World War II. An explosion of mustard gas left American sailors with extremely low white blood cell counts. When this news reached physicians who were treating leukemia patients (typically with exceptionally high white cell counts) it triggered research into the possibility of using the chemical components of mustard gas to wage war against leukemia. As a result, leukemia became the first cancer to be treated with chemicals and thus chemotherapy was born.

Today the chemotherapy of choice for ovarian cancer is usually a combination of Taxol and another chemical with a platinum base. I was told I would receive Taxol, which is a drug extracted from the bark of the Pacific Yew tree, and Carboplatin. Carboplatin binds with the DNA of cancer cells thus preventing their reproduction. Taxol is said to actually cause cancer cells to become temporarily inactive, allowing the Carboplatin to move in for the kill.

My friend Maureen Burrill (who goes by the nickname Corky) had gone through chemotherapy following breast cancer four years previously. Corky not only gave me encouragement and hope, she insisted I needed to go outside of Kaiser for a second opinion. Since this was a constant refrain I'd also heard from numerous other friends, I agreed. Corky recommended her own oncologist, made an appointment for me, and then even drove me to UCLA in West Los Angeles for the appointment. I was extremely grateful for her help and support and thrilled to have a personal guide through the maze of offices at the UCLA Medical Center.

Corky and I met with Dr. William Isacoff. He'd had a chance to review copies of all my records from Kaiser that I'd mailed to him, and we discussed my proposed chemotherapy. After careful consideration of all the treatment possibilities, Dr. Isacoff said he believed I could probably forego the chemotherapy altogether since I had no evidence of cancer outside the ovary. He then agreed that Taxol and Carboplatin were the drugs he would recommend should I decide to go ahead with chemotherapy.

Encouraged that my HMO was offering the same treatment suggested by UCLA's team of experts, I scheduled another appointment with Dr. Chang and told him Dr. Isacoff's opinion. But Dr. Chang held firm. He said I could probably do a less extensive program than the eight treatments Dr. Semrad had ordered, but because I'd had an atypical clear cell carcinoma, he wanted me to undergo chemotherapy, at least four treatments.

My next stop was Dr. Semrad's office. I told him my second opinion had recommended no chemotherapy. Dr. Chang had suggested four treatments. Dr. Semrad insisted I go all the way with eight treatments. Three respected physicians had given me three different opinions, and I was naïve enough to think that this was unusual. I would later learn that much of what researchers know about cancer treatment via chemotherapy is still in the embryonic stage.

Chemotherapy may not remain as a first-line treatment along with surgery and radiation therapy in the future, but at the time of my cancer experience, chemotherapy was the best available treatment. I would wait a few more weeks for my incision to heal completely and to regain my strength before treatment would begin. Theoretically the chemotherapy would kill any remaining cancer cells in my body, but in order to do so many healthy cells—besides the obvious hair follicles—would also die. These powerful chemicals could track down and destroy even microscopic cancer, before the cells could regroup into another tumor and possibly kill me.

The focus of my life now shifted to preparing myself physically and mentally for a procedure that could be as life threatening as the disease itself.

The Wellness Community

I had to wait for my incision to heal completely before I could begin chemotherapy. During this time, I returned to the breast cancer support group and explained my current status. None of these women had ovarian cancer, but they all had experienced the feelings of what it's like to hear the diagnosis of cancer, feelings that are unknown to "civilians," as we liked to call those who have never had cancer. Cancer was something we shared and I know their hearts went out to me. Every member of the group hugged me and wished me well. They all promised to call me while I was going through chemotherapy.

I walked out of the meeting actually feeling hopeful, but then the group facilitator pulled me aside and asked if she could have a word with me. We stepped into a vacant meeting room and she closed the door. She spoke very gently, but she explained that the breast cancer group was no longer right for me. She said that I should find another support group, one that was open to people with multiple cancers.

I didn't understand, so I pressed her for an explanation. Her gaze dropped to the floor and became riveted there, as if something really fascinating was going on between her feet and mine. She finally admitted that my presence in the group was threatening. My unusual case was simply too frightening for the other breast cancer patients to handle. They might become overly apprehensive that another primary cancer could show up in their bodies as well.

Her words went through me like a low voltage shock. I was being cast out of a group that was supposed to be a necessary part of my recovery. I suddenly realized why Sandy, the woman who'd developed colon cancer shortly after her breast cancer, had never returned to the group. My eyes were moist, but anger rose in my throat just the same. I was pretty much speechless which was definitely unusual for me.

When I questioned her request, she said I had to think about the others. They would live in fear of developing ovarian cancer themselves just by my presence in the group. I was guilty as charged I suppose, tainted by not only breast cancer, but the dreaded killer ovarian cancer as well.

My normal fighting spirit was daunted. What logical argument could I possibly present? My anger dwindled into a hurt no less than a stab wound to the heart. What choice did I have but to retreat like a common social outcast?

My positive attitude had taken a nosedive. Perhaps I should have stormed the office of the hospital's medical director, demanding reinstatement, insisting that I should be an exception to this unthinkable policy, but my heart simply wasn't in it. Here I was about to undergo a treatment possibly worse than the disease, and I had lost my connection to the friends who had helped me make peace with the breast cancer. Of course I could still talk to these women on the phone, but I knew it just wouldn't be the same.

I'd read that Dr. David Spiegel, a Stanford University psychiatrist, had conducted studies between 1985 and 1993 in which he established that women attending breast cancer support groups had a significantly longer survival rate than those who did not participate in a group (37 months versus 19 months). Dr. Spiegel described his research in his 1994 book, <u>Living Beyond Limits: New Hope and Help for Facing Life-Threatening Illness</u>. It had been documented. I decided I needed another group.

I thought back to the weeks immediately following the mastectomy and remembered a lovely woman from the American Cancer Society who had visited my home as part of the Reach to Recovery program. Esty Lohnberg was a breast cancer survivor herself, and in addition to sharing her cancer story with me, she had given me a soft cotton temporary breast form that I could tuck inside my bra until

I'd healed sufficiently to be fitted for a prosthesis. She'd also given me a packet of information containing lists of resources for cancer patients. I searched for those lists and came upon the telephone number of The Wellness Community.

I'd heard good things about The Wellness Community, and I also remembered how Gilda Radner had praised the group in her book. Dr. Harold H. Benjamin, a former attorney, founded The Wellness Community in 1982 after his wife was diagnosed with breast cancer. It is a non-profit organization that offers an incredible array of services to people with cancer and their families, all at no cost. It is the largest psychological and social support program of its kind in the United States. (Incidentally, Harriet Benjamin is still alive!)

Dr. Benjamin started The Wellness Community with one facility in Santa Monica, California, and has since expanded to facilities throughout the country. I called The Wellness Community in Westlake Village, the location closest to my home, and made an appointment to attend an orientation meeting.

I was expecting to see dozens of people at this meeting, but I was the only person attending besides the facilitator, a pleasant, caring woman named Anne Gessert. We talked, but mostly Anne asked me questions. At first I was cautious, thinking I was being screened for objectionable qualities, like having too many different kinds of cancer, but this was not the case at all.

The main purpose of the orientation, as I saw it, was to explain that belonging to one of The Wellness Community support groups required a commitment. Anne asked me to attend at least three meetings before making any decision to withdraw, should I decide to do so. Once committed, I was expected to attend every week unless I was ill or away on vacation. This sounded okay with me, so I signed up for the Thursday morning participant group. While I met with others who had cancer, Morrie would meet in the next room with the spouses, parents, or significant caregivers of my group members.

At the first meeting I told everyone my cancer story. We all had a story, and telling it was part of the process. Cancer patients share many experiences, such as chemotherapy, even if the cancer itself is different. It was great to be able to talk about something as alien as chemotherapy and to feel normal doing so. In fact, The Wellness Community was the only place I felt "normal" regarding a lot of things during this frightening period of my life.

We willingly shared many practical ideas, like taking a tape recorder along to our medical appointments because we would frequently be overwhelmed by the vast array of information the doctor would present to us regarding proposed treatments or upcoming surgery. We also learned to make a list of all the questions we wanted to ask our doctors in advance of appointments. These were little things, but I saw at once that by sharing ideas, we gained strength.

At the first few meetings I didn't volunteer very much, partially because I was new, but also because I was still a little gun shy after being asked to leave the breast cancer support group. I soon learned, however, that my apprehensions were groundless. I became a part of the group and stayed an active member for more than two years.

I still marvel at the early days. I didn't think it was possible to walk into a room filled with total strangers and immediately feel surrounded with love. It was as if our souls had met. We laughed. We cried. We told each other our fears, and in doing so, the power that fear held over us just seemed to melt away. Eventually, as a group, we came together in complete understanding.

Our group facilitator was a wonderful woman named Maryana Palmer. She was a licensed psychotherapist who took the lead when someone faltered, but mostly she just encouraged us to say what we really felt and to give our love and support freely and openly to one another. The sense of feeling connected to the group was a very powerful medicine. Just learning that someone with a similar diagnosis has recovered boosts your own recovery. Likewise, being able to give comfort to someone who is worse off provides far-reaching benefits to both.

No amount of money could buy what I got from my support group. The other cancer patients gave me understanding rather than pity. By sharing information and experiences, my sense of control was enhanced. Suddenly I no longer felt alone in my fight against cancer, and the warmth of being part of such a closely-knit group made it easier for me to cope with my fears.

At The Wellness Community we crushed many of the myths about cancer that seemed to prevail almost everywhere, and as we chased away the cancer boogiemen, we made a real effort to change our own mental attitudes.

I became friendly with many brave survivors at The Wellness Community, but I grew especially close to Ginny Baker, a nurse who had leukemia, and Barbara Foerster, a retired hospital dietitian. Barbara also had ovarian cancer, so we bonded immediately, eagerly exchanging notes about the deadly monster that had invaded our bodies.

Barbara's stage III ovarian cancer had been diagnosed in October 1994. For more than a year prior to that time, she'd seen various doctors because of diarrhea/constipation, gas, and intermittent pain. They didn't find anything more serious than what they believed to be an irritable bowel syndrome. Barbara didn't know about the CA 125 test, and apparently her internist didn't think of it either. All those months while she was being treated for irritable bowel syndrome, ovarian cancer had spread throughout her peritoneal cavity, with omentum, bowel, vaginal, diaphragm, appendix, and cervical metastases. By the time a CA 125 was finally administered, her count was up to 6,800. Normal is 0-35.

When I met her, Barbara had been having one form of chemotherapy or another nonstop for a year and a half. You would've thought that all of this chemotherapy on top of an inaccurate diagnosis would've left Barbara in a really foul mood. Not a chance. I can't recall ever seeing Barbara when she didn't have a radiant smile on her face and kind words for every one she spoke to.

Each of us at The Wellness Community had his or her own unique set of circumstances. We had lung cancer, breast cancer, ovarian cancer, brain cancer, esophageal cancer, leukemia, melanoma, multiple myeloma, and cancer of the thyroid. There were differences, yet there was always a common thread running within the group.

Someone would make a statement about an uncomfortable or frightening feeling that had surfaced during treatment or surgery, and three others would chime in, "Yes, yes. That's what it was like for me, too."

The men and women in the group talked about things that we never would have discussed with "civilians." We told each other about fears and feelings that we wouldn't even tell our husbands or wives.

Sexual dysfunction was a common concern because chemotherapy often sends sexual desire into a tailspin. The women who did not have ovarian cancer joked about their ovaries being "fried" by the drugs, birth control via industrial-strength toxins. Then too, if a woman isn't already in menopause, chemotherapy will sometimes bring about its onset, instantly, no matter what her age. We discussed the sudden loss of sexual desire, vaginal dryness, and hot flashes while the men in the group nodded sympathetically. They were having problems of their own trying to sustain an erection or reach orgasm because of decreased sensation resulting from chemotherapy.

We learned to discuss everything, even those subjects that were traditionally taboo in polite company. Many of the group participants found that if they mentioned their fear of dying to a family member they were immediately hushed.

"Don't worry. You're going to be just fine."

"You're not going to die."

"Now, now, dear. Let's not talk about that. Would you like some chicken soup?"

The denial was meant to ease the patient's fear I'm sure, but the subject of death was one that needed to be discussed in our group. At The Wellness Community we had that opportunity, and no one hushed us for trying to come to terms with our own mortality. We talked about death—or more specifically the pain of dying that is often associated with cancer. Once we realized that this was a universal fear, and that it was okay to be afraid, the fear usually slipped away.

Those in the group who had cancer in its advanced stages worked overtime trying to get the most out of life. They traveled and they had fun, both life-affirming acts, but they also reached out to others in the group. The love and genuine caring for one another was unbelievable.

Barbara especially treasured every moment, calling each new day her "bonus time." But Barbara was not living in a state of denial. She knew she would eventually die from her cancer. She acknowledged that death is simply a part of life, and coming to terms with death made each day of her life more rewarding.

Barbara's dependence on chemotherapy in order to extend her life, much like a diabetic depends on insulin, meant she would never be able to reclaim her pre-cancer good health. Instead, she found ways to adapt to living with cancer, rather than denying it. Barbara had been struck down but not destroyed. She proved to all of us who live under the shadow of this disease that we could maintain patience and contentment in our lives in spite of cancer.

Thanks to Barbara's wisdom and judicious guidance, I was able to accept the reality that like everyone else, someday I would die. Once I'd shed the fear of death, I was ready to live. By helping the members of the group come to terms with death, Barbara became stronger. We all became stronger.

We also grew to understand that the fear of death is a negative emotion and to want to live is a positive one. We never referred to ourselves as "victims" of cancer. Emphatically, we were all cancer survivors! We learned that we should never believe there was nothing left to do in our fight against cancer. There is always hope for those who believe that hope is an actual factor in dealing with the disease.

Before our own diagnoses, many of us had known people who had died of cancer, but most of us didn't know <u>anyone</u> who had survived it. It was important to get together to learn about recoveries, remarkable ones as well as the predictable. In short, we, as a group, came to believe that we all could recover, and holding that conviction of wellness deep in our hearts was every bit as important as our medical treatments.

Even those with seriously advanced stages of cancer were encouraged not to give up. We all knew cancer treatments did not come with guarantees, but we all agreed to fight for recovery, enjoying life to the fullest along the way.

Climbing Mt. Everest

On May 16, 1996, I celebrated my 55th birthday. Just two weeks post surgery, I wasn't able to do much more than sit on the sofa. Six close friends came by with dinner and loads of wonderful gifts for me, and we spent a quiet evening at home.

Later, when I studied the snapshots Morrie had taken that night, I discovered that I'd aged from undergoing four major surgeries in such a brief period of time. I looked hollow-eyed and extremely tired. After the ovarian surgery especially, everything I did was a monumental effort. I had absolutely no energy.

The following week my dear friend Pamela Jordan Schiffer flew in from Baltimore to visit. I was delighted to see her, but I couldn't help worrying that she had gone to the expense of flying all the way to California simply because she equated my ovarian cancer with certain death. It was difficult to get that thought out of my mind because many of my other friends had worn a decidedly concerned look on their faces when they'd heard about my second round of cancer.

So many women don't survive ovarian cancer, that some of my friends seemed convinced I <u>couldn't</u> survive it. Every time I told someone I had ovarian cancer, they looked terribly distressed, making me feel as if I already had one foot in the grave. Of course there were others who didn't look at me that way. I reasoned that perhaps they were doing their best to keep up a happy front just as I knew Morrie was doing. Friends from all over continued to call or visit and it was hard for me not to wonder what they were really thinking. I guess my over-active writer's imagination was trying to craft a demented story out of all of this, and thankfully my neurotic phase didn't last too long.

By the end of May, Dr. Chang believed I was strong enough to begin chemotherapy. In preparation, Morrie took me to a wig shop where I bought three wigs in my natural hair color, dark brown with a hint of gray. I tried on a long, blond Dolly Parton wig, but somehow it just wasn't me. Morrie confirmed this when he simply couldn't stop laughing.

I went into the hospital for blood work a few days prior to the first chemotherapy treatment. When I was finished in the lab, a nurse took me into the chemotherapy room and explained the procedure that I would follow. Along the windowed wall of a long narrow room stood about a dozen chairs similar to the kind most dentists use. At that moment, several reclining patients were hooked up to IV apparatus. Most were alone, but one woman had a man sitting close to her. He looked worried enough to be her husband. They didn't look too happy, but then again they didn't look entirely miserable either.

Along the opposite wall I could see several doors leading to individual patient treatment rooms. Each tiny room had a hospital bed and its own private lavatory. Since my regimen would require anywhere from six to eight hours of continual IV drip, I would receive treatment in one of the private rooms.

The nurse then set up a video for me to watch that would explain the side effects of chemotherapy. After a nurse on camera had discussed the management of nausea, a vivacious-looking woman with a full head of beautiful curly red hair came on the screen. The redhead explained that most chemotherapy patients lose all their hair. She displayed a collection of close-fitting hats, scarves, and turbans that, according to her, would surely brighten up any outfit.

In a few short minutes I had grown to hate this perky young woman who was happily chattering about the many ways a colorful scarf covering my soon-to-be-bald head could boost my spirits. I wanted to do some serious damage to this video. Before I had a chance to disgrace myself, however, the redhead reached up and yanked off all those

41

bouncy red curls in one grand sweep. It was a wig! The woman didn't have a hair—red or any other color—to her name. I guessed this was a new form of shock therapy.

The nurse then gave me a folder of information and instructions regarding chemotherapy. I also received a prescription for steroids in pill form that I would begin taking the evening before each treatment. The steroids were supposed to help me tolerate the chemotherapy, and to insure that I had an adequate level in my body, I even had to set the alarm and swallow tablets during the night.

Treatment number one was scheduled a few days later. In the meantime I had my hair cut to a <u>very</u> short style. This move was supposed to make my hair loss seem less traumatic.

On the day of my first treatment, I arrived at the chemotherapy room at 8 AM, ready, but very nervous. I wondered how the toxic chemicals would feel as they dripped into my veins. I tried to shake the anxiety growing in the pit of my stomach, but it didn't budge an inch. That morning my blood pressure was higher than it's ever been in my life, but the nurse said that was quite common with first-time chemotherapy patients. She smiled and took me into one of the private treatment rooms and started an IV.

The first drip contained something to hydrate my veins and a sedative to relax me. This seemed like a logical approach considering how wired I felt. Next, I received Decadron, another steroid, again to help me tolerate the Taxol. Then came a bag of Benadryl, an antihistamine used to help prevent allergic reactions to the chemicals I was about to receive, and a bag containing an antibiotic. Each bag dripped slowly into a vein in my left hand, and thus the entire morning was spent allowing these four drugs to set the scene for the highly toxic cancer killers yet to come.

Morrie and Nancy were with me the entire time all this was going on. Nancy sat cross-legged on the foot of my bed cheerfully joking with the nurses and talking non-stop. It didn't take an expert to figure out that she was trying to distract me from the reality of what was actually happening.

What she said didn't matter. A black hole had formed in the center of my mind, and just having Morrie and Nancy in the room helped me fight the overwhelming desire to close my eyes and simply pass out.

We didn't know it at the time, but while Nancy waited patiently in hospital corridors or sat on my bed amusing me during chemotherapy, a seed was germinating in her mind. The dedicated nurses who had cared for me inspired Nancy to enter the nursing profession. She would soon finish college and then enter nursing school, going all the way for her degree and RN license. Nurses are exceptional individuals and it later made complete sense to me that Nancy would follow this path.

I became very drowsy during the hours of chemotherapy but never fell completely asleep, mostly because the nurses were very attentive, constantly monitoring everything they could possibly monitor. An aide came into my room and asked me what I would like to order for lunch. He handed me a printed menu from the hospital's dietitian.

The nurse whispered, "Order the thing you like the least."

I ordered a turkey sandwich and then asked the nurse why she recommended something I wouldn't especially like.

She grinned and then explained that during chemotherapy strange things can happen to your taste buds. Foods I loved could become immediately offensive and then I might develop a total aversion to that same food which could last indefinitely. I'd never loved turkey sandwiches, so this would not be a great loss, but I stored that bit of information away for my next treatment.

Meanwhile the nurse began my Taxol drip. A sensation of fiery heat coursed up my left arm and seemed to make my arm feel heavier than normal. In moments I began to feel warm all over, as if I had developed a sudden fever. I felt the beginning of a headache and I started to feel sick to my stomach at the same time. The nausea subsided after a few minutes, but the headache pounded away at my frontal lobes for the rest of the day. Right about this time, Dr. Chang came

43

in to see how I was doing. He assured me that the procedure was going well, and I seemed to be tolerating the Taxol without any perceptible difficulty.

I noticed that when the nurse handled this particular chemical, she wore protective gloves and goggles, something she hadn't bothered to do with the steroid or the antihistamine. Putting myself completely in someone else's hands like this suddenly left me with an overpowering sensation of helplessness, especially with such toxic chemicals dripping into my bloodstream.

I was allowed to get up to go to the bathroom, towing my IV equipment along with me, but I was told I should flush the toilet twice after each use and scrub my hands thoroughly with hot, soapy water. A sign to this effect—printed in very large, black letters—hung in the lavatory in case I forgot. I was also instructed that it was necessary for me to continue this same meticulous hand scrubbing and double flushing routine when I got home.

Then the nurse explained the procedure I needed to follow regarding my toothbrush. First, I was cautioned not to allow anyone else in the household to even touch the toothbrush that I would use for the next seventy-two hours. At the end of the three-day period, I was ordered to drop my contaminated toothbrush into a plastic bag, seal the bag securely with tape, and throw it into the trash.

I was groggy, but not so sedated that I didn't understand the gravity of these precautions. Protective gear for the nurse, double-flushing of my bodily excretions, unprecedented hand-scrubbing, handling my toothbrush like a venomous reptile? Any minute I expected a haz-mat team to come in and carry me away in a lead-lined receptacle. The realization that the poisons flowing into my body were even more toxic than I'd previously thought finally hit home.

I was given the Taxol and Carboplatin along with Zofran, a drug that relieves nausea. The day seemed endless. With their usual thoughtfulness, Scott and his wife Ellen had given me a Sony Walkman cassette player for my birthday. I managed to get through the hours of infusion by listening to guided visualization and imagery on tape. I listened to two tapes over and over: "Chemotherapy" recorded by Belleruth Naparstek for Time Warner Audio Books and "Relaxation and Guided Imagery" recorded by Harold H. Benjamin, PHD, for The Wellness Community.

With visualization I created a mental picture that represented my fight against the cancer similar to Dr. Simonton's methods. There are no right or wrongs to this mental process. Some patients imagine white knights in armor slaying dragon-like cancer cells while others think of a rocket or bomb blasting the cancer to kingdom come. I visualized the chemotherapy that was dashing through my veins as a sleek silver chariot delivering the magic needed to kill any rebellious cancer cells that may have gone underground to hide out somewhere in my body.

I'm certain that if anyone from my mother's generation knew that I was trying to ward off additional cancer with a tiny imaginary chariot, I would've been directed to the nearest mental institution, but there is increasing evidence that these techniques have a valid place in cancer treatment.

If nothing else, visualization can relieve stress and give you a feeling of "doing" something positive. While I was lying there with my entire body being infused with chemicals that were too noxious to even touch, my life seemed anything but in my control. The doctors and nurses were doing their best to eradicate the cancer, but I needed to be a part of this process. I believed that any activity in which I felt the slightest degree of control was a step in the right direction.

I also listened to "Love, Medicine & Miracles" recorded by Dr. Bernie S. Siegel for Harper Audio Books and his words were extremely encouraging and soothing.

At the end of what seemed like an eternity, I was disconnected from the last IV tube. Somehow, I walked out of the medical center with Nancy half-holding me up. Morrie had driven the car right to the hospital door, but I didn't think I could walk the incredible distance to the curb. The feeling of being more intensely fatigued than I'd ever been in my life was the only thought that entered my mind. I felt like a punctured tire.

I don't remember the ride home, but I remember facing the stairway that leads from our living room to the second floor. It had become a monumental challenge, and I doubted I was up for it. The strength had gone out of my legs. My knees felt rubbery. I couldn't focus on anything except how difficult it was to place one foot in front of the other. Getting upstairs and into bed was like climbing Mt. Everest.

Bald Isn't Beautiful

Aside from the fatigue, the most unpleasant side effects from the chemotherapy did not appear in full until the day after treatment. Then came the ripples of nausea, which in my case wasn't as bad as I'd expected, and the pain, which was much worse. I'd been told that the chemicals would probably cause muscle aches and neuropathy (nerve damage causing pain and numbness), and both of these predictions came true. Pain seeped everywhere. Even the soles of my feet ached, and combined with the neuropathy in my legs, it was difficult for me to stand or walk for any length of time.

Every muscle in my body seemed to be throbbing. I didn't know how my body could survive this internal assault. I knew that anything powerful enough to kill cancer cells would also have harmful effects on my healthy cells, but I wasn't prepared for the daggers of pain that sliced through my muscle tissue. Morrie and Nancy fussed over me, bringing me food and medication or wiping my face with a cold washcloth, but basically I just wanted to be left alone.

My hands were too shaky to sign my name on a check, so I couldn't pay bills or even keep up with correspondence. My eyes didn't focus well enough to read, write, or watch TV, so I was back in bed listening to my tapes. After a few days, I realized that I needed to go beyond the step of visualizing the chemotherapy chariot delivering magic treatment to my cancer cells. Again with help from Linda Ruhle, I began using guided imagery to try to bring about a change in my overall health for the long term as well as trying to relieve the pain at the moment.

Guided imagery is actually a form of daydreaming. In my mind's eye, I tried to envision myself in perfect health. Linda taught me to think of cancerous cells like cubes of sugar dropped in water, dissolving away. I visualized myself graciously giving up any anger that I may have been harboring regarding the cancer. I gave up thinking that I might die. All negativity had to go. I became so specific in my thinking that I decided to make a tape of my own, so I could lead myself through the various steps of my mental excursion following the sound of my own voice.

When I used my personalized tape, I went into our bedroom and closed the door. At first Morrie came racing into the room, I guess fearing that I was slashing my wrists. When he realized what I was doing, a closed door then designated that no one was allowed to disturb me. He took phone messages; the house was generally very quiet.

On the worst days, I would lie on the bed, but when I felt able, I sat on a rocking chair, my feet flat on the floor. I closed my eyes and took several deep breaths before I started the tape. My hands rested on my knees; my back was straight.

I had incorporated breathing instructions into my tape, so I wouldn't forget to take long, full breaths during the entire time I was following the course of my imagery adventure. With each breath, I imagined I was inflating a large balloon in my stomach, causing my stomach to rise. This forced me to breathe deeper than normal. After a few more deep breaths, I began to methodically relax my body, starting with my head and neck and working down to my toes. When I reached my toes, I imagined all disease, pain, and fatigue sinking down into the floor and plummeting straight into the earth below where it would disappear forever. Some people recommend starting the relaxation process with your feet and working up, but I don't think it matters as long as you achieve total relaxation. Personally, I liked the idea of plunging all the negative stuff in my life deep down into the earth.

I then began to imagine myself as completely well. I was centering all my energy, all my positive thinking in one direction: getting well. Sure, I was following the plan of treatment devised by my doctors, but I was also treating myself with good, healthy energy created from my own thinking. I believe there is a remarkable connection between the mind and body, and the guided imagery was a powerful form of medication. I _expected_ positive results. I truly believed I would get well, and I didn't give in to any more thinking about dying.

Many instances have been documented where a placebo worked to actually cure a disease against all odds simply because the patient _believed_ the remedy would be successful. In the same vein, a positive belief system (without so much as a placebo) is also a powerful healer. The conscious belief has to come first, and then that hope will be transmitted to the body's healing system and immune system. Believing— truly believing—I would get well helped my body to fight the disease right along with helping me cope with the treatment itself.

Next, I imagined myself doing what I wanted to do most, which was to continue with my writing career. I'd had two mystery novels and many short stories published prior to the cancer, but now I was having trouble signing my own name. I pulled up images of myself back at the keyboard, hard at work. I envisioned myself in New York receiving a prestigious national award, like the Edgar for best mystery novel, in front of hundreds of cheering authors and editors. I walked up to the podium to receive my well-deserved award looking slim, gorgeous, and _healthy_ in a knock out designer dress. (As long as it was my positive thinking at work, I figured I'd go all the way.)

By the sixth day following the chemotherapy, the pain had subsided but I was noticing great clumps of hair—even though it was short hair— stuck in my comb. I stopped combing altogether, but the hair continued to fall. I now had wide noticeable bald patches all over my head, so I returned to the hair salon. Chris Lavine, my hair stylist, shaved off all my hair, and with each swipe of her electric razor, I came closer and closer to tears. By the time she was finished, Chris had tears in her eyes also. She refused any payment for shaving my head and I quickly put on the wig I'd carried in with me and hurried out of the salon. I cried all the way home.

Eleven days after my first chemotherapy treatment, I did not have a single hair anywhere on my body. The loss of hair, clinically known as alopecia, is total. To a woman who hasn't experienced hair loss, it is difficult to explain just how devastating it can be. I went to The Wellness Community and shared my feelings. I wasn't the only woman in the group wearing a wig or a hat, so they understood. Amelia Prince, Barbara Foerster, Maria Alvarez, and Irene Woolley were also hairless from chemotherapy. No one ever mentioned the fact that my hair would grow back. We all knew that. Hair growing <u>back</u> wasn't the point.

The point was that I felt even more depressed over losing my hair than I'd felt over losing my breast. The missing breast was replaced by my prosthesis, and it was easy to dress in such a way that no one would ever suspect I'd lost a breast. Not so with hair loss. I felt too unnerved to go bald, so I wore a wig everywhere except in the shower. At first I didn't even want Morrie to see my baldness, but I came to realize that he loved me no matter how awful I looked. He reassured me at least a hundred times that my getting well was all that really mattered.

At night I slept in a soft cotton turban. I even avoided looking at my hairless self in the mirror. I penciled in eyebrows to help conceal the blank look on my face that resulted from the missing eyebrows. I wore sunglasses whenever I went outdoors because I had no eyelashes. I felt that my femininity had taken a real beating, so I made certain I <u>always</u> wore lipstick and earrings, just in case a strong wind came up and blew off my wig. I know it sounds crazy, but somehow the feminine embellishments helped me to feel a little more secure.

Added to the loss of my breast and reproductive organs, this additional loss was brutal. I listened to my personal guided imagery tape three or more times a day. I felt like <u>The Little Engine That Could</u> repeating, "I think I can. I know I can," over and over. I said my affirmations aloud. I said them silently. I kept trying to substitute positive, supportive statements for all the negative ones that popped into my mind whenever I looked in a mirror. These affirmations had a powerful effect on my body as well as my mind. I had to get well. Heaven probably requires a photo ID, and I was bald.

As the days passed, my group at The Wellness Community became even more important to me. Irene, Maria, Amelia, Barbara, and I exchanged notes about problems associated with being hairless. I learned to use a special shampoo, Nioxin, on my bald scalp rather than the bar of soap I used on the rest of my body. Nioxin prevented one of the common plagues of chemotherapy, dandruff as big as corn flakes. No new information about anything ever got by us. We shared everything.

Sharron Goldstein, who was also undergoing Taxol chemotherapy for ovarian cancer, had just joined our group and frequently went au natural because wigs and hats made her feel too hot. I admired her spunk and freedom, and I have to admit that on her bald was beautiful.

Four weeks had passed since my first chemotherapy treatment, and the pain had finally faded. Although I was still very tired all the time, I was so encouraged by this comeback that we scheduled a two-week trip to Scotland with my sister and her husband, Betty and John Morrisson, for August. Dr. Chang assured me that he could schedule my chemotherapy so we could leave on our trip exactly two weeks after one treatment, returning a day or two before the next.

Looking forward to Scotland was helping me to cope, but just when I was finally feeling much better, I realized it was time to face treatment number two.

Chemo Brain

The first chemotherapy session had damaged a lot more than my hair follicles. Blood tests revealed that my red blood cell hemoglobin count had fallen beneath four grams. A normal count is twelve to sixteen grams. Below eight grams anemia occurs, so that explained why I was always so tired. I also had a reduced number of white blood cells, a condition that makes it difficult for the body to fight off infection, and a reduced number of platelets. When the platelet count falls, the blood does not clot easily, so I had to be careful not to cut myself.

I'd lost lymph nodes from under my right arm and my pelvic area. This, combined with low blood counts, left me a walking, talking candidate for more life-threatening infection. Since I had to avoid cuts and burns, Morrie banished me from the kitchen. If I did accidentally cut myself, I had to remember to take care of it immediately. I used tubes of antibiotic creams almost as freely as hand lotion, and I always had at least one Band-Aid adhesive strip somewhere on my right hand. I was told that I needed to wear gloves when doing anything like gardening, so Morrie declared that for me yard work and house cleaning was out of the question. I was beginning to see that even cancer has a few advantages.

In order to avoid a very painful condition called lymphedema, I had to remember to have all medical injections, blood tests, and blood pressure readings done only on my left arm where I still had lymph nodes. Lymphedema involves severe swelling of the arm as a result of blocked, damaged, or missing lymph nodes.

I was also warned to avoid professional manicures because infections are sometimes spread via shared equipment. I even had to avoid wearing tight elastic cuffs around my right wrist.

All of these precautions had become a necessary part of my daily existence and would remain so for the rest of my life. With this level of constant vigilance over so many little details, I knew it would be impossible for me to ever forget that I'd had cancer.

Cancer can be a hard-hitting wake-up call. I did not believe that my life was over by a long shot, but I also now realized it could be over in a minute. Something about having cancer makes you suddenly a lot smarter. I understood that in life we do not get a dress rehearsal. I remembered to exercise all the cautions.

I checked in for my second chemotherapy treatment early on a Friday morning in June. The procedure was very much the same, except this time I was armed with a gigantic bag of Reese's Peanut Butter Cups. Peanut butter cups have always been a real weakness with me, so I'd decided to try aversion therapy compliments of the chemotherapy in hopes of developing a severe loathing of my favorite candy.

I couldn't take more than two bites of my turkey sandwich. The sandwich just didn't appeal to me, so I began eating peanut butter cups. I started out slowly. They tasted great. I continued to eat one peanut butter cup after another. No aversion developed, but by the time I'd consumed half the bag, I realized I was on the road to making myself sick, not to mention fat, if I didn't stop. I tossed the rest into the trash. The aversion therapy didn't work, and suicide by peanut butter cups clearly was not the answer either. Go figure. To this day, I still love peanut butter cups, but I hate turkey sandwiches.

This time I staggered out of the hospital with Nancy supporting my right arm, and my stepdaughter Deborah holding me up on the left. Just walking a very short distance was like trying to climb a waterfall.

The side effects of Taxol and Carboplatin are cumulative, so the pain, nausea, and general discomfort of the second treatment were more severe than the first time around, especially the pain. Again I ached everywhere. If I'd had a hair on my head, I was certain it also would have been aching. I was back in bed, this time understanding that I would be there for the next week to ten days.

Again, after three days, I had to seal my toothbrush in a plastic bag and discard it. I drank gallons of water to flush the chemicals out of my system and to maintain proper kidney function. We scheduled nothing other than getting through each day one day at a time. Every evening I prayed for the energy and stamina to keep the positive energy flowing through my mind and body.

It was right around my second chemotherapy treatment when I realized that Morrie seemed to be taking my illness even harder than I was. When I was so terribly sick and weakened by the intense pain in my muscles and joints, I took pain pills and went to bed. I was often too sedated to do anything other than sleep. Many times while I slept through my pain, Morrie would sit in the rocking chair in our bedroom, silently watching me and worrying. I was certain it wasn't merely a coincidence that his hair was rapidly turning gray.

On the worst days when I wasn't sleeping, I listened to my tapes. Many cancer patients will swear that guided imagery reduces pain. I don't know how much my pain was actually alleviated, but I did enjoy a deep feeling of serenity and soothing restfulness. The relaxation combined with imagery tended to clear my mind of any negative thoughts that tried to work their way into my thinking.

When I could read, I read books about how other people had overcome cancer. My friend Mary Johnson had given me a copy of <u>Remarkable Recovery</u> by Caryle Hirshberg and Marc Ian Barasch, and I savored the accounts of these incredible recoveries little by little each day. The starch had gone out of me physically, but I also realized I was having trouble concentrating. Reading a book took me a long time. My mind used to be sharp, but now details slipped through it like a free-flowing sieve. Names of people and places and other details that I had known without question for years and years suddenly went flying right out of my head. It was positively frightening.

As soon as I could, I returned to The Wellness Community. Again, we exchanged notes on the side effects of chemotherapy. It was helpful to know that I wasn't simply being a big baby regarding my reactions to the Taxol. Reactions vary from person to person. Give ten people the same chemotherapy, and to one degree or another, each will be affected differently. And just in case we weren't already depressed, we were told that some chemotherapy regimens actually cause a form of clinical depression.

Many of my friends in the group had tolerated their chemotherapy better than I had, but they were not all on Taxol. Two women had reactions to Taxol that were so severe, they could not continue taking the drug. Barbara Foerster had to be hospitalized for six days following her first and only treatment of Taxol and Carboplatin. Her doctors decided to give her less debilitating drugs for subsequent treatment.

During my chemotherapy The Wellness Community was not only helpful, it was indispensable. Being with other cancer patients provided me with a feeling of normalcy that somehow had disappeared from my life along with the diagnosis.

Group assurance was necessary for all phases of what was happening to me. I was reluctant to mention that my concentration was weak and my memory had apparently turned to oatmeal, but I finally owned up and shared this embarrassing bit of information.

"I know just what you mean," Barbara said. "I've been calling myself 'Chemo Brain' for months."

"I thought I was the only one," Maria cried.

We all laughed at ourselves, again happy in the knowledge that no matter how awful things seemed, we were not alone.

We learned to think of our healing process as a daily task, something that doesn't automatically happen overnight.

We discovered there are no short cuts. You have to take the steps to recovery one at a time. We often felt like lab rats running a maze. I'd received three differing opinions from three different oncologists, and when other members of the group reported similar experiences, we all became less fearful about the many uncertainties we faced.

There was always someone in the group going through chemotherapy. We shared our concerns about the drugs, but we also discussed our personal fears regarding treatment. Chemotherapy had a way of forcing our deepest feelings and anxieties to float to the surface.

We talked about the future, about the dreams and hopes we wished for ourselves, but mostly for our families. Men and women alike worried about how their families would cope if the cancer were victorious, but it was also universal that we all had positive hope for a miracle.

Somehow we helped each other to endure the rigors of chemotherapy. Whenever a member of the group announced a positive reduction in tumor size, we cheered and hollered like a bunch of crazed football fans at the Super Bowl.

Then Lloyd Isham joined our group after being diagnosed with a terminal brain tumor, and Irene Woolley reported that her lung cancer had metastasized to her spine.

Some days we felt like we were trying to build a fortress out of cooked spaghetti, but we shared a saying that I think was first attributed to Eleanor Roosevelt: "When you get to the end of your rope, tie a knot in it and hang on."

Thought I'd Die Laughing

A man walked into the vet's office carrying an obviously sick dog. "Can you tell me what's wrong with him?" the man asked.

The vet placed the dog on a table and looked at him. Then the vet left the room, returning a few minutes later with a cat. The cat slowly walked a complete circle around the sick dog and then turned and circled around the other way.

The vet said, "I'll have to keep your dog overnight. So far your bill is two-hundred and fifty dollars."

"What for?" the man shouted in disbelief.

"Fifty dollars for the office visit and two-hundred for the CAT scan."

A diagnosis of cancer does not mean you have to lose all pleasure and happiness in life. Maintaining a sense of humor might be the best medicine of all. At The Wellness Community we laughed at jokes a lot cornier than the one above. If a joke had anything to do with doctors or the medical field in general, it would usually find its way into our weekly support group meeting.

A doctor told his patient, "I have bad news and worse news."

"What's the bad news?"

"You have cancer."

"Well, what's the worse news?"

The doctor said, "You have Alzheimer's."

"Oh, good, at least it's not cancer."

All the many times I met with my support group, Morrie was in the next room meeting with family members of the participants in my group. Occasionally, during their intensely sorrowful sessions, they would hear a rousing roar of laughter emanate from our room. Morrie and the others were always amazed that while <u>we</u> were the ones with cancer, we seemed to be having a much better time than our caregivers.

We encouraged each other to have as much fun as possible. After our group sessions each week, many of us went out to lunch together, along with our spouses, as a further extension of the friendships we'd formed. We invaded a favorite local deli and shared a wonderful esprit de corps along with our food. It was also a chance for me to become better acquainted with the husbands and wives of my friends in the group. When we were together, we constantly cracked jokes, and I always laughed loudest when the joke was on me.

The Wellness Community even held an annual joke fest. We got together with no other purpose than to tell jokes and have fun. Dr. Terry Paulson, a volunteer coordinator at The Wellness Community and internationally known speaker, always served as our master of ceremonies. The jokes were so incredibly bad we couldn't help laughing, and our laughter was always contagious. Many of us laughed until our sides ached, and then we laughed some more. We discovered early on that while we were telling jokes and laughing until we cried, thoughts and worries about cancer fell by the wayside.

With chemotherapy destroying our red blood cells, we were all exhausted most of the time. One day Maryana Palmer, our group facilitator, announced that The Wellness Community was hosting a guest speaker who would discuss ways to manage our fatigue. She suggested that hearing this information might be helpful, but we all quipped that we were much too tired to attend a lecture on fatigue. (A few of us went anyway.)

It didn't take long for me to discover that kidding around with my doctors helped to relieve a lot of my fears. I also suspect that a bit of humor might reduce some of the stress our overworked medical champions must experience in the course of dealing with patients who are often scared to death in addition to being critically ill. For example, when Dr. Schilling explained to me that my breast lumpectomy would be performed on an outpatient basis, Morrie and I both registered surprise. At first I couldn't believe they were actually going to send me home on the same day of major surgery.

I thought about this for a moment and then said, "I guess I should be grateful Kaiser doesn't have a drive-up window."

Dr. Schilling laughed, and we laughed along with her. Morrie later said that it was just like me to turn something like cancer into a series of one-liners.

In other words, I believed it was important not to let "life" come to a halt while I was fighting the cancer. One day Barbara Foerster said cancer had taken years out of her life, but it wasn't going to take life out of her years. We all subscribed to that thinking.

Having cancer is hard work, and dealing with doctors, treatments, and various medical procedures can literally consume all the patient's time and energy. The idea is to live as full a life as possible while undergoing all the tests, scans, and chemotherapy. Coping with unfamiliar medical challenges can sap what's left of one's strength, so it's important not to let go of the child within you. We learned to permit that child to seek out and participate in as much fun as possible.

We all agreed that if we had a choice of videos to rent or movies to watch on TV, we would select a comedy. We rented the Marx Brothers or Abbott and Costello. It didn't matter that we had already seen many of these timeless films; the important thing was to put everything into the proper perspective and make fun a top priority in our lives. I discovered television classics on cable and spent many happy hours enjoying "I Love Lucy" reruns all over again. The wrinkles we get from laughing are much better than the ones we get from sulking and worrying. Perhaps Victor Hugo expressed it best when he said, "Laughter is the sun that drives winter from the human face."

When friends asked us what they could do for us, we suggested that the friend find something humorous for us to read. It didn't matter whether it was a novel, a joke book, or a collection of cartoons, just so it was something that tickled our funny bones.

The movie "Patch Adams" starring Robin Williams brought to light the need for a daily dose of humor for seriously ill patients. The real Dr. Hunter D. "Patch" Adams of West Virginia firmly believes in the restorative powers of humor. He has traveled to places like the bleak pediatric wards in Russia and Serbian refugee camps in Bosnia wearing a clown suit and a bulbous red nose. Dressed in his clown costume, he dispenses laughs rather than pills in order to comfort sick and dying children.

Research has shown that after a good laugh, your blood pressure is lowered, your heart rate drops, your muscles relax, your body stops producing cortisol (a hormone associated with stress), and you feel an increased sense of physical and emotional well being. Sounds like a better deal than taking medication to achieve the same results.

Then one day someone came into The Wellness Community with this story:

When a man walked into the doctor's office, the receptionist asked him what he had.

"Shingles," the man replied.

She told him to take a seat and fifteen minutes later a nurse came out and asked him what he had.

He said, "Shingles."

The nurse took him into an examination room and took his blood pressure and his temperature. She told him to take off his clothes and put on a hospital gown.

A half-hour later the doctor came in and asked him what he had.

"Shingles."

"Where?" the doctor asked.

The man said, "Outside in the truck. Where do you want them?"

Laughter can be hazardous to cancer. I tried to remember any jokes I'd heard recently. It was time for my third round of chemotherapy.

Friends

My third chemotherapy treatment went pretty much the same as the first two, except this time school was out for the summer and four close friends from my teaching days were now on their summer break. Ruth Baker, Betty Rabin Fung, Relda Blythe and Jonna Barr wedged into my tiny treatment room along with Morrie and Nancy.

I was so groggy from the medications that it was hard for me to feel upbeat, but my friends insisted on turning the seven-hour ordeal into a party-like atmosphere. We shared gossip and told jokes. They made me laugh even as the toxic chemicals dripped into my veins.

I was grateful to have the love and friendship of my former colleagues in my little chamber of horrors. In spite of the warning signs regarding double flushing and hand washing and the haz-mat accouterments of the nurses, my friends somehow understood that supportive relationships were necessary and even beneficial to my healing. Coming in the wake of another friend completely turning her back on me because I had cancer, their support was especially crucial to my recovery.

Cancer is a disease that most people find terrifying. Nowadays almost everyone has lost a friend or loved one to cancer, but for the most part, there is a serious lack of accurate information about cancer among the general population. Many people feel inadequate when they come up against a serious illness of any sort, but with cancer, and now possibly AIDS as well, that feeling of helplessness is further magnified by a kind of mythology surrounding these diseases. Most of these myths, of course, are completely untrue. Cancer is not a curse—it's simply a terrible disease that manages to frighten people into doing things they might not ordinarily do.

The woman who had abandoned me completely—I'll call her Alice, not her real name—had been my friend ever since we were kids in junior high. We'd shared the intense joys and agonies of our teenage years, telling each other everything. When it came to our dreams and desires and even our plans for the future, we had no secrets. Alice and I went to dances and parties together. We listened to each other's records by Elvis Presley, The Four Lads, and Pat Boone. When she wasn't at my house, I was at hers, usually watching Dick Clark's "American Bandstand" on television.

Alice lives in another state now, but we'd kept in touch by phone and wrote letters over the years. I knew our mutual friends had informed her that I'd hit the daily double with two cancers, but I hadn't heard from her at all, not even a get-well card.

I assumed that Alice was afraid to call because she didn't know what to say. Many people freeze up when talking to cancer patients, fearful that they'll say the wrong thing, when simple words like, "I'm thinking about you," would be enough.

But with Alice too much time had gone by. The more I thought about it, the more I began to worry about _her_. Perhaps something terrible was going on in her life, and she didn't want to worry me. Maybe she was afraid that I was doomed to die, and by keeping her distance she could avoid the heartache of losing a friend. All sorts of crazy things went through my mind. I decided to call her.

My attempt at mending fences with Alice failed miserably. She said, no, there was nothing terrible going on in her life at the moment, but hearing about my cancer had apparently hit too close to home. She'd lost a family member to cancer in the past, and now, to avoid facing her own fears, she simply had to avoid me.

I was devastated. I hadn't asked her to become involved with the ups and downs of my treatment. I certainly hadn't asked her to visit. I simply wanted my old friend to still care about me. Maintaining social contacts was important to me, and I couldn't understand why she wanted to push me out of her heart so completely. I wanted to be treated the same as before my diagnosis. I was the same person; I'd been a good friend, and now I felt cheated.

I realized there was nothing I could do to change the way Alice felt. For whatever reasons, she was not willing to go through this illness with me. I wondered if all cancer patients had someone like "Alice" in their lives. I hoped not. I now understood that a true friend is one who walks in when others walk out. Friends couldn't make my treatment any easier, but having them rally around me as they did during that third round of chemotherapy was a blessing I'll never forget.

I went home from the medical center that evening feeling incredibly weak. I literally crawled up Mt. Everest and fell into bed. I was disoriented. Our bedroom light was too bright; barely audible sounds were too loud. I couldn't think. I felt completely defenseless against the poisons running through my bloodstream. My skull felt too small for my throbbing brain. I slept fitfully, waking every few hours even though my fatigue had not diminished.

The next day the ever-increasing cumulative effects of the chemotherapy began to pummel my muscle tissue. By evening I ached everywhere I had a muscle and a few places I didn't know muscles existed. Even my teeth felt achy. Then the one muscle I hadn't previously thought about initiated a violent protest to the chemotherapy.

My heart had suddenly begun hammering out of control.

Deadly Side Effects

In <u>Gilda's Disease</u>, Dr. Piver points out that less than one percent of women given Taxol for ovarian cancer will develop a serious irregular heart beat from the chemical. It figured that I would be a member of that small, select group.

I waited for the rapid pounding of my heart to slow down. It didn't. My heartbeat seemed to fill the room, perhaps the entire house. It definitely filled my head. I couldn't hear anything over the runaway thundering of my heart. I was certain the arrhythmia couldn't possibly last even another second, but my heart continued slamming hard against my ribs, raising my level of anxiety with every resonant thump.

I sat down with a book and tried to ignore the arrhythmia. Naturally, that didn't work. I was afraid to tell Morrie what I was thinking because I didn't want him to panic, but I began to fear that I was actually going to have a heart attack and die.

My heart continued pounding. I became so terrified I had to tell Morrie what was happening to me. It seemed there was no end to the pain and worry I was causing him. He looked stricken, but he took control of the situation in that determined but gentle way of his.

In moments, we were on our way to emergency.

By the time they had me hooked up to an electrocardiogram, I felt as if I were holding on by a very thin thread. Everything had flipped out of control and I was growing more apprehensive by the minute. I was feeling dizzy and my heart simply would not slow down; each beat conjured up visions of a heart attack. I was given medication, but my heart rate continued at an alarming 184 beats per minute.

After a few hours my condition was regarded as stable even though the arrhythmia continued. Gradually the severe thrashing of my heart muscles subsided to a very rapid but more regular pulse. But even as my pounding heart slowed, it was still beating twenty percent faster than normal. I was finally sent home and told to rest.

It took another two days before my heart rate returned to what felt like my normal rhythm. My nerves had been frazzled from this whole experience, but I gradually regained a sense of composure. I scheduled an appointment with Dr. Chang to review these most recent and frightening side effects of the chemotherapy. He just sighed and nodded in sympathy when I told him about the arrhythmia and my trip to emergency. He explained that there simply is no way to accurately predict how the toxic chemicals used in chemotherapy can affect a patient. Each person has to be treated on an individual basis.

"Can you be certain I won't have a heart attack if I continue with the chemo?" I asked.

"No," he answered.

I went to see Dr. Semrad and asked him the same question. Again, the doctor offered me no guarantees. Dr. Semrad wanted me to have more chemotherapy just to be on the safe side in dealing with all the unknowns surrounding the clear cell carcinoma, but he said he certainly would understand if I should decide to discontinue treatment. Whether I continued or not, he said, was up to me.

I went home and did some serious thinking. I kept coming back to the same question. Did I want to die of recurring cancer or from a heart attack? The whole thing seemed ludicrous. How was I supposed to know what to do? More chemotherapy would surely set off the terrifying arrhythmia of my heart once again. On the other hand, quitting chemotherapy could cost me my life. I had three weeks to make my decision, and less than one week to pack for our trip to Scotland.

As with all my cancer issues, I took my dilemma to The Wellness Community. This was not an easy call, but then we didn't participate in a support group simply to have someone else make decisions for us. We discussed my options. We discussed how important it is for the cancer patient to take part in his or her own recovery. I was not only taking part, at the moment I was in full control and I was scared to death. We also discussed how my quality of life might be altered if the chemotherapy actually triggered a heart condition that was not fatal.

I left the group that day without having resolved my problem, but I felt as if I'd received permission to make my decision without fear of criticism. Everyone was rooting for me to make the correct choice. Now all I had to do was figure out what the correct choice should be.

Iona Abbey

Focusing on our upcoming trip to Scotland helped me to shift my thinking away from the decision I had to make regarding the chemotherapy. The trip would be a welcome release from the many months of surgery, antibiotic infusion, and chemotherapy I'd just experienced. My sister Betty Morrisson and her husband John had been my most important source of strength and familial love during the forty or so years they'd been married. Both are steadfast, caring individuals but also full of fun. I knew we would have a wonderful time in Scotland, but as anxious as I was to spend two weeks with my sister and brother-in-law, I wondered if I'd have enough strength to keep up with the others on the tour.

It took me about four days just to assemble and pack my clothes. I would place a few items in my suitcase, and then I'd have to stop and rest. I'd go back to the closet, locate a few more essentials, and then I'd need a nap. I was still bald, so I packed an extra wig in addition to the one I would wear, just in case. (I was certain Scotland would have strong, gusting winds whistling across the moors.) Little by little, I gathered everything we would need.

When we finally departed I was still suffering from the fatigue of anemia, but sheer determination kept me on track. When Morrie and I arrived in London I was exhausted after the long flight, but thrilled to see Betty and John who'd arrived from their home in Virginia a few hours before us. We talked non-stop over dinner that first night in London and then fell into our beds, dead tired but in high spirits. We boarded the bus for Scotland the following morning.

We spent a few glorious days seeing the sights in Edinburgh, including the annual Edinburgh Military Tattoo, perhaps the world's best known and most loved military spectacular. The color and lights and the music of hundreds of pipers and drums filled the esplanade of Edinburgh Castle with a dazzling, magical performance.

After Edinburgh, we traveled north. Once we'd reached the northernmost point along the eastern coast, we ferried off the mainland of Scotland to the Orkney Islands. We visited Skara Brae, the ruins of a Neolithic village dating back to 2,500 B.C. and the Ring of Brodgar, the Stonehenge of Scotland, which, like its counterpart on the Salisbury Plain in England, is surrounded by an aura of mystery.

We then traveled west to delightful villages across the highlands. The craggy landscape of northern Scotland seemed to be home to many more sheep than people. Since Scotland is located just south of the Arctic Circle, the summer days stretched late into evening. After dinner in the slowly fading daylight, we wandered along the docks of fishing villages or the streets of quaint old towns where the sturdy little homes were crafted out of the same rugged stone as the countryside.

It was almost like traveling back in time to a more peaceful, gentler era. We were a long way from telephones, computers, and television sets, and I was delighted that we had the opportunity to share this experience with Betty and John. We were free to walk and meditate in silence, or we could spend time talking and reminiscing.

Morrie and John usually walked at a faster pace than I could handle, and I knew Morrie wanted a chance to spend time alone with my brother-in-law. Morrie cherished the friendship that had grown over the years between the two of them, and he undoubtedly unloaded some of his own fears about my cancer on John's shoulders. Fortunately, John was there for him just as Betty was there for me.

Betty and I trailed behind them, quietly exchanging memories. Although my sister had telephoned me at least once a week during the previous eight months to offer her love and support, this was the first chance we'd had to talk in person about my cancer. I shared my fears and explained the choice I would have to make regarding continuation of the chemotherapy. The first week of our trip had already passed and I was still struggling with this dilemma. As soon as we returned home, I would have to make my decision. Similar to the members of my support group, Betty didn't tell me what to do. While I rambled on, she listened, nodding and encouraging me to follow my instincts.

I also confided to Betty that it was not simply a question of how quitting chemotherapy could shorten my life. I had to consider the quality of life I would have if I developed a serious heart ailment. Even as I said it, I remembered that the term "quality of life" was regarded as a euphemism among cancer patients when they become aware that very little "quantity" of life remains.

We traveled all the way to the windswept western coast of Scotland, which is dotted with many islands called the Hebrides. From the little town of Oban our tour bus boarded a ferry to the island of Mull. Then the bus bumped along, over winding country roads, transporting us across Mull. Occasionally our driver had to stop and wait patiently while a shepherd directed his flock of sheep across the road in front of us. The narrow roads finally brought us to the tip of a long, slender peninsula that jutted out like an old woman's finger, pointing to the west. From this extremity, we left the bus behind and went aboard a much smaller ferry that transported only foot traffic, no vehicles, to the tiny, treeless island of Iona.

My close friend Mildred Darby, the former librarian at the junior high school where I had taught English, had visited the island of Iona numerous times. It was through Mildred that I'd first learned of Iona's magical qualities. This speck of land—one mile by three and a half miles—is home to the Iona Abbey that played a major role in bringing Christianity to Britain. Today the Iona community is an ecumenical religious group that maintains the Abbey much as it was back in the thirteenth century.

Iona Abbey has been celebrated for centuries as a focal point of spiritual energy, and thousands of pilgrims visit the stark stone building on the high and windy cliffs of Iona each year. Once inside the Abbey, I could feel the powerful force of the presence of a higher being even though the Christian trappings within the building had nothing to do with my own Jewish faith. Nevertheless, a surge of rarefied spirituality was definitely there, and I was surrounded by dynamics I couldn't explain. I had experienced these inexplicable waves of energy only once before in my life. That had been almost ten years earlier at the Western Wall of Solomon's Temple in Jerusalem.

I approached a recessed altar that was lined with dozens of flickering votive candles. Other visitors quietly meandered about exploring the abbey, but I stood there completely mesmerized. I seemed to be alone in the abbey, somehow blocking everyone else from sight and mind. My concentration was so deep, I felt as if I were the only person on the entire island. I finally picked up a taper and lit a candle myself. It seemed like a perfectly natural thing for me to do even though I had never lit a candle in a Christian religious setting before in my life.

I stood at the little altar, hypnotized by the glowing candles and filled with the intensity of a force I couldn't see. I silently prayed for the wisdom and strength to make the right decision regarding my chemotherapy. I prayed for guidance. I prayed for a continual flow of positive energy to keep me going through the weeks and months to come.

It was that simple. Suddenly, without any fanfare, I was no longer torn in two directions. I knew exactly what I had to do. The Scottish saints had somehow given me the insight that I could get well and stay that way but only if I stopped permitting my medical team to pump deadly poison into my veins.

Linda Ruhle had taught me that self-healing is directly connected to one's thinking. Just as I believed that my mind held power over my body, I now knew that prayer was a vital component of this same dynamic force.

My prayers rang in my ears. The healing energy of Iona Abbey had permeated my soul. I was no longer discouraged, apprehensive about my decision, or even tired. I suddenly possessed more energy than I'd had in months. I knew my positive thinking was being transmitted to my immune system. Occasionally a tiny corner of my intellect surfaced with questions about the wisdom of my unexpected epiphany. I had to set aside any doubts; I had to believe I was making the right decision. I forced myself to suspend the impulse to revert to my former more traditional way of thinking.

I wasn't quite ready to admit to others exactly <u>how</u> I'd reached my decision, but I now believed that I could safely discontinue chemotherapy and still beat the cancer. The "What if I'm making a big mistake?" question simply faded from my mind.

I told Morrie and Betty and John what I had decided, but I didn't tell them about my sudden insight into the whole problem until much later. I had never been more certain that I was making the correct choice than I was at that moment.

After Iona we had a few more days of travel before we were scheduled to fly home. Except for the fact that John became very ill with a serious viral infection the last two days of the trip, the whole experience was wonderful. I'd communicated with my only sibling on an intimate level that I don't think we'd ever reached before, and as a result, we'd bonded even closer.

And on a tiny island thousands of miles from my home, I'd found the inner strength to make perhaps the most difficult decision of my life.

On My Own

Morrie was very supportive of my decision to quit chemotherapy, but then I knew I could always count on him to back me no matter what. I wasn't so sure I'd get the same kind of endorsement from Dr. Chang and Dr. Semrad.

Dr. Chang was very understanding and didn't argue with my decision, although we did discuss the possibility that the ovarian cancer could recur simply because I hadn't been able to tolerate the chemotherapy. He made certain I understood the chance I was taking. I didn't bother to mention that I'd made a pilgrimage to an abbey in a very remote corner of the world and that I now had a whole army of Scottish saints in my corner. I believed some things were best kept to myself.

Dr. Semrad tended to lean toward the more scientific approach. He explained that Taxol had been clinically tested using eight or more rounds of treatment. Treating a patient with only three rounds such as I had received had never been studied. He said I might be making a mistake, but he certainly didn't want me to continue the chemotherapy if I was fearful of damage to my heart. The look on his face, however, revealed that he was far from comfortable with my decision.

Word got around. The next time I went in for a routine check-up, I overheard two of the young doctors who were working under Dr. Semrad talking about me. One said to the other as he pointed me out, "She's the one who quit chemotherapy."

Some of my civilian friends were shocked that I'd taken matters into my own hands. In spite of their apprehension, I stuck with my decision. One thing I'd learned from my support group at The Wellness Community was that it's always easier to let the medical experts make decisions for you. But by relinquishing all decision making, the patient's power also is given over to the doctors. By acting on her own behalf, the patient takes a giant step toward getting well.

My friends at The Wellness Community understood this perfectly. They not only supported my decision, but they also congratulated me for taking an active role in my own recovery. I understood the chance I was taking, but I also believed I would remain cancer free even though the statistics may have been stacked against me. I was determined not to let a fear of the unknown take over my life.

My euphoria regarding my decision to stop chemotherapy did not last long, however. There was certainly nothing scientific about my decision, and in fact, I sometimes wondered if my "religious" awakening in Iona Abbey had been nothing more than a moment of temporary insanity. I'd traveled a long way from the spot halfway around the globe that had given me so much confidence, and it was somewhat unsettling to realize that I was now on my own.

I'd entered into a twilight zone of sorts, and at times I couldn't help feeling uneasy. I'd heard other members of my support group talk about the feelings of insecurity that had arisen when their respective treatments had come to an end.

"Suddenly you feel alone and unprotected, like you're off somewhere in limbo," they would explain, "but mostly there's this feeling that no one is 'doing' anything to help you fight the cancer."

As horrendous as chemotherapy had been for me, I had to admit it had served as a security blanket of sorts, helping me to face the disease. But I'd opted to recover without additional chemotherapy, so I made up my mind to explore other avenues. Naturally, I would continue to have routine medical checkups by both surgeons and my oncologist, but their job would be to "catch" a possible recurrence of the cancer. My job would be a bit more involved. I had to subscribe to a lifestyle and a mental outlook that would "prevent" a return of the disease.

Just about the time I'd reached all these conclusions, I got a telephone call from Irene Woolley. She'd been receiving radiation treatments for the lung cancer that had metastasized to her spine so she hadn't been to The Wellness Community for several weeks. She reported that she had fallen—trying to get to the bathroom—and broken her hip. She was in a hospital about 20 miles from my home, and as soon as I hung up the phone, Morrie and I were on our way.

When we walked into her hospital room, I was shocked to see the undeniable changes in her appearance. The radiation and the cancer had taken a severe toll. Her once-lovely eyes had sunk deep into her ashen face, and her usual cheerful smile couldn't be called up no matter how hard she tried.

Someone had left a tray of food sitting in front of Irene, but she didn't have the strength to pick up the fork. I fed her cubes of Jell-O and a few mouthfuls of mashed potatoes, but it was difficult for her to swallow. She told me she'd had hip surgery and she would be sent home in a day or so. I thought that was odd, thinking she'd need at least a week or two of physical therapy for the hip, but then it registered. They were sending her home to die.

I made two trips to Irene's home the following week. By this time she was unconscious and groaning in pain. A long-time friend of Irene's had traveled from San Diego to be by her side. This genuinely concerned woman took me aside and told me how she'd spent the entire night praying for Irene's recovery. I explained as gently as I could that I had done just the opposite. In its advanced stages, cancer is tough to eradicate. I knew that Irene's disease had won, and I had prayed for her pain to be over quickly. Irene died the following morning.

I met the same woman again a few days later at Irene's funeral. She said I'd been right and she asked me how I'd known that Irene would not recover. Like so many others in our society, Irene's friend knew almost nothing about cancer. She'd heard stories that incorporated a few of the myths surrounding the disease, but her knowledge stopped there. I hardly knew what to tell the poor woman.

Irene had been one of the unlucky ones. She was my first friend from The Wellness Community that I'd lost. Unfortunately she wouldn't be the last.

Although I didn't recognize it until much later, a unique part of my life was unfolding, my healing journey.

Reaching Out

I was beginning to get the message about cancer: Rotten things definitely can happen to good people. I was starting to wonder whether there was anything the average layman could do to make a difference. I wanted to reach out to people like Irene, to actually "do" something positive to help, but I sure didn't know what.

As for me, I wasn't fully recovered from the chemotherapy. My blood counts had improved somewhat but remained below normal. I still had no hair, but my overall stamina had improved slightly. I knew my body was healing, but the process was extremely slow.

I decided to call the American Cancer Society in response to a letter I'd received from them asking for volunteers. I felt I was well enough to help the ACS in some minor capacity, providing the task was not too strenuous. They had a perfect job lined up for me.

Along with a few other breast cancer survivors, I was assigned to work at a post outside the entrance to one of our local supermarkets. We talked to women entering the store and explained the importance of routine mammograms. Along with our pitch, we passed out information regarding low-cost mammograms at a nearby clinic.

Sounded like an easy day, but I was dumfounded by the number of women who readily admitted they'd never had a mammogram. One woman claimed that if she had breast cancer she didn't want to know about it. She said she was quite content to be blissfully ignorant of any cancer that may have invaded her body. We gave many women the address of the clinic that was offering the low-cost mammograms, but those women who refused to even hear the facts terrified all of us.

I had been on duty for several hours and was getting ready to go home when a woman came over to me. Blandette Bush introduced herself and confided that she'd recently been diagnosed with breast cancer. We chatted for a long time and made arrangements for her to stop by my home so we could talk some more. Blandette clearly needed a friend at this point, and we hit it off immediately.

When she arrived at my home we discussed the options her surgeon had presented. She had been given the choice of lumpectomy or mastectomy with very little information to guide her in making a decision. I shared my many books with her, and we talked for hours. Blandette is extremely intelligent and logical, so she recognized the benefits of my positive thinking theory and adopted it as her own.

I even bared my chest and showed her what a mastectomy looked like. I also gave her the soft cotton "first" prosthesis that Esty Lohnberg from Reach to Recovery had given me. This helped to further ease her fears, and in the end she elected to go for the full mastectomy as well. We agreed to go through our cancer days together.

Blandette was taking a medical leave from her job at IBM, so I encouraged her to become involved with The Wellness Community. She immediately joined a support group, though not the same one that I attended. Together we also discovered a very special group of women called the Westlake Village "ABC" Support Group who meet once a month at a local hospital.

ABC, which stands for After Breast Cancer, was founded in 1984 when a handful of breast cancer survivors got together simply to provide support for one another. The group's membership has since expanded and this extraordinary organization now serves hundreds of breast cancer survivors in our community by providing educational services as well as many activities that are arranged strictly for fun. The American Cancer Society has recognized and commended ABC for its programs and the emotional support it provides for women. Bonded by the traumatic experience of breast cancer, these women become instant sisters. I can think of no stronger affiliation.

Since then Blandette and I have attended dozens of informational meetings at The Wellness Community as well as ABC. At ABC we met and became friends with Toni Domenic, and the three of us took advantage of the many parties, potluck dinners, and exercise classes these organizations provide for people recovering from cancer. My close relationship with Blandette and Toni made a big difference in my recovery. The laughter we shared replenished my soul, but we also cared for each other, encouraging one another to enjoy and appreciate every moment.

Each year ABC, in conjunction with the American Cancer Society, also conducts a class called "Look Good, Feel Better." Special makeup tips are provided for women going through chemotherapy (such as using sunscreen where our eyebrows used to be) plus hints regarding effective ways to cope with hair loss.

We especially enjoyed attending Saturday morning Chi Gong (Qigong) classes at The Wellness Community. Chi Gong is an ancient Chinese healing technique that combines very gentle physical movements with meditation and rhythmic breathing.

Tina Rollo from my support group was always cheerful and spunky in spite of her breast cancer, and she frequently joined Blandette and me for Chi Gong. Tina was the most industrious (and successful) real estate salesperson I've ever known, and she continued to sell houses long after she was diagnosed. She often stopped by her real estate office in order to deliver escrow papers or set up a termite inspection on her way home from one of our classes.

Since we all had low blood counts, none of us had enough stamina to participate in anything like an aerobics class, so Chi Gong was a perfect exercise session for the three of us. We worked hard at perfecting the slow, precise movements, and we actually became quite good at releasing and directing our chi (the body's vital energy) to all the right places in our bodies. Releasing our vital energy promoted the healing process, and we left our morning sessions feeling calm and relaxed, but somehow at the same time we felt marvelously energized.

Every spring ABC holds a fashion show featuring fashions for women who've had breast surgery, and every June The Wellness Community hosts its annual "Day of Celebration" for cancer survivors. Hundreds of people participate in both of these activities every year. The Day of Celebration includes an enormous barbecue, live music, and arts and crafts projects for cancer survivors' children and grandchildren.

One year my granddaughter Maddie de Channes, who was eight at the time, accompanied me, and she enjoyed having her face painted by an artistic clown. The clown transformed Maddie into a happy-faced dog with floppy ears and a lolling tongue. Everyone applauded Maddie's puppy-like smile and her willingness to be such a good sport. Maddie's good-natured spirit made her an instant hit with all my friends.

Blandette and I also ran—well, actually we walked—in the American Cancer Society's Relay for Life. The event raises money for cancer related programs while it gives survivors a chance to pass the word on to others. We felt like soldiers, taking up arms against this unwelcome disease, as we proudly joined other cancer survivors in executing the first lap around our local high school track.

Shortly after Blandette and I became friends, I met Linda Blaustein, a survivor of ovarian cancer. I was unable to convince Linda to take advantage of a support group or any of the other services at The Wellness Community, but nevertheless we became cancer "buddies." We had countless sessions on the phone, discussing our cancer treatments, but we also spent many pleasant afternoons engaged in what we called "shopping therapy." Linda also introduced me to "Conversations!" a newsletter published for those fighting ovarian cancer by a tireless woman from Texas named Cindy H. Melancon. (CHMelancon@aol.com)

Back in 1993 Cindy felt very isolated during her chemotherapy, so she tried to contact other women facing the same battle. It took her seven months to locate just one other woman with the same kind of ovarian cancer. With no money, no experience, and no equipment, she then launched her first newsletter, sending it to only ten women with ovarian cancer. Four years later, Cindy had 1200 on her mailing list from all fifty states and five other countries.

Since then Cindy has converted most of her home into a spectacular resource center for women who are fighting the disease. With no financial support other than the scattered donations she receives from fellow survivors, she has established a non-profit organization devoted entirely to educating and helping women cope with ovarian cancer.

By the summer of 1995, Cindy and Gail Hayward, an ovarian cancer survivor from Florida, had formed the basis of what later became the National Ovarian Cancer Coalition. They saw a need for a national awareness group and a need to make enough noise to expose the "Silent Killer" as the enemy it is. All this evolved because of Cindy's driving need to connect with other women who were combating the same cancer. Our government could learn a lot by observing the dedication and enthusiasm of people like Cindy Melancon.

Thanks also to efforts by Cindy and Gail and other persevering women, the Ovarian Cancer National Alliance's First Advocacy Conference was held in Washington, DC in September of 1998. The OCNA is the umbrella organization that coordinates activities nationwide in an effort to make some serious progress regarding ovarian cancer issues. That same month, President Bill Clinton proclaimed a week as Ovarian Cancer Awareness Week. We have since been elevated to an Ovarian Cancer Awareness Month. A small step forward for ovarian cancer perhaps, but forward motion nonetheless.

I also joined the National Breast Cancer Coalition, a grassroots organization that fosters breast cancer advocacy. Breast cancer activists from across the nation work with the NBCC, hoping to make a difference. Their main focus is lobbying lawmakers in Washington, DC for financial support for breast cancer research. They also work to improve access to high-quality screening, diagnosis, treatment, and follow-up care for all women, but particularly for low-income women who have little or no health insurance and therefore are more likely to die from breast cancer because of delays in diagnosis.

Almost a year had gone by since my first diagnosis and by this time I'd learned to live one day at a time. My life had been returned to me, and I realized I had to regard each day as a new and precious gift. I was not the same person I was before cancer, and I now know that I will never be the same. I doubt that anyone walks away from cancer untouched, and I've learned from many of my cancer "buddies" that cancer can leave you a stronger, better person.

Yet at the same time, no matter how positive he or she tries to be, the cancer survivor always has the fear of recurrence hovering somewhere in the background like a persistent bad dream. Even for those who survive, this fear does not go away completely. I kept trying to convince myself that my positive thinking, the visual imagery, and my prayers were all that I needed, but none of this is as easy as it sounds.

My oncologist never uses the word "cured" for a reason. Cancer treatment does not come with a guarantee. Cells from a tumor can lie quietly for many years and then suddenly regroup, or a new mutation can emerge therefore bringing about an entirely new cancer. At times it is almost like waiting for the other shoe to drop.

Nonetheless, I clung to the statistics for reassurance: According to the American Cancer Society, forty to fifty percent of people who get cancer will recover from the disease. Eight million Americans have survived cancer, at least three million for five years or more. Many of the three million are considered fully recovered. I was trying to carve a safe little niche of my own within those three million.

Fighting a Dismal Battle

By November of 1996, I had been wearing a wig every day for almost six months. Five of those months I'd been completely bald, but by the sixth, I'd begun to grow a bit of fuzz on my scalp. Although most people didn't even realize I was wearing one, my wig was hot and annoying and I could hardly wait to be rid if it. One day I took a peek at something we had roasting in the oven and the heat that escaped singed off the acrylic bangs from one of my wigs!

I frequently spoke to Maria Alvarez from my support group on the phone, and she, too, was finally seeing the fuzzy new growth of her hair. Maria was a petite fifty-year-old with beautiful dark, expressive eyes. Maria smiled easily, but she didn't just smile, she glowed. She had a very gentle nature, and I was drawn to her as a friend. Before her breast cancer, Maria had worked many years as a nurse at the UCLA Medical Center. Now she was a patient there.

Maria mostly wore cute knitted hats that suited her more than a wig, but hats can be hot and uncomfortable, too. Comparing notes about our little tufts of hair usually sent us into giggles just like a couple of kids. We finally decided that we would "come out" together and planned to go to the next meeting of our support group sporting only our marine-style crew cuts. With barely a half-inch of hair on our heads, we were feeling great, and that day our positive attitudes reached a new high. All of our friends at The Wellness Community loved our new look, and we felt pretty proud of ourselves.

Maria's oncologist had concluded that her type of breast cancer was at a very high risk for recurrence, so she'd had a stem cell transplant performed a few months earlier to provide her with the optimum chance of recovery.

Stem cells are manufactured in the bone marrow, and they give birth to platelets as well as red and white blood cells. During a traditional chemotherapy regime such as I had received, the drugs will usually annihilate the body's stem cells. If all goes according to plan, however, the bone marrow will recover in due course and then resume its production of these vital cells. The stem cell transplant, on the other hand, makes it possible for the patient to receive chemotherapy at increased levels that otherwise would possibly kill him or her.

Maria's stem cells were harvested from her blood prior to the transplant using an intricate blood-separating machine. The collected stem cells were then set aside and carefully frozen. Following this fairly effortless harvesting procedure, Maria then received several concentrated rounds of extremely toxic chemotherapy.

Maria had been well aware that 10 percent of stem cell transplant recipients die during the process, not from their tumors, but from the rigorous treatment itself. Maria also knew that her immune system would be severely compromised by the high doses of cancer-killing drugs, but she took the risk in order to live. She described the concentrated chemotherapy as grueling, and at times she'd felt so sick she almost wished she were dead. After a few days of this intensive drug infusion, the harvested stem cells were taken out of storage and gradually returned to her blood. The returned stem cells were then able to grow into new blood cells and literally "rescue" Maria from possible death from the devastating effects of the chemotherapy.

Maria went through this horrendous procedure twice, with only a short break between treatments. As with traditional chemotherapy, the patient must wait to see what happens next. If the cancer did not return within five years, Maria would be able to rest a bit easier. If the cancer never came back, only then would she know that her stem cell transplant had been a complete success.

Maria didn't have a very long period of remission. After a few short months she'd begun to experience body pain. A tumor marker test for breast cancer indicated her cancer had returned. The test, the CA 2729, measures proteins manufactured by breast cancer much the same as the CA 125 measures proteins given off by ovarian cancer. CT and bone scans of her entire body then revealed metastatic tumors in her bones, the largest in her collarbone.

Maria had been given such massive doses of chemotherapy during the stem cell procedure that she dreaded the prospect of returning to the sea of waiting rooms, doctors, and medical procedures she thought she no longer needed. She began radiation treatments directed to the tumors growing in her bones. She also eventually resumed weekly chemotherapy but at a lower, more user-friendly dosage.

Maria's prognosis was frightening. Sometimes a doctor's dire prediction can work as a hex on a person's chances of recovery, but Maria was not discouraged. She had no intentions of giving up her fight for recovery, but she also confided to me that she was very much aware that her life would never again be the same. The fear of dying in unbearable pain, which is usually a more persistent fear than death itself, was one of her greatest concerns as the pain in her bones intensified.

I was feeling dismal about the thought of losing my friend Maria. In fact a few of my civilian friends wondered why I made an effort to maintain close friendships with my group members who were undoubtedly going to die from their cancer. Wasn't it hard enough to lose family and other long-time friends without going searching for new friends who wouldn't be my friends for very long?

I thought about Maria, struggling with breast cancer, as well as Barbara Foerster and Sharron Goldstein, suffering from advanced stages of ovarian cancer, and the answer became simple. Having their friendship and love, however briefly, was a phenomenal gift, one that I would not have traded for all the peace of mind in the world.

Soy Milk, Tofu, and Green Tea

I was gradually getting back into the routine of cooking (although Morrie still watched me like a hawk whenever I ventured near the stove), and along the way I'd read numerous articles and a few books about the connection between healthy eating and cancer prevention. Every time I picked up a newspaper I'd notice another claim. The experts all had different theories, and the confusion was enough to send me out in search of a Big Mac and fries from Mac Donald's.

Dr. Harry Menco, an oncologist at the Los Robles Regional Medical Center in Thousand Oaks, spoke about the issue at an informal gathering of breast cancer survivors. He discussed a famous study of Japanese women that had concluded there was a lower incidence of breast cancer in Japan than America because Japanese people eat less fat than we do. The study showed that once a Japanese woman moves to the United States and takes up our fat-laden fast food habits, her breast cancer risk then equals that of any other American woman.

But, according to Dr. Menco, more recent research has proven that the lower rate of cancer is not because Japanese women don't eat fat, but rather because they do eat large quantities of soy. Since this most recent study was published, newspapers, magazines, and even talk shows have jumped on the soy bandwagon.

In a position paper presented at UCLA, David Huber, Ph.D., Director of the UCLA Center for Human Nutrition, acknowledged that soy may "inhibit cancer growth." The National Cancer Institute (NCI) is currently investigating the use of soy as a cancer preventative because soybeans are reputed to contain a number of anti-carcinogens (substances that prevent cancer growth).

Additional claims by researchers contend that adding soy products to the diet enhances the immune system thereby preventing the growth of some cancers. Genistein, one of the isoflavones found in soy, is supposed to slow angiogenesis (development of blood vessels that feed tumors) and cause cancer cells to return to normal cell status. When I read that only one serving per day of soy may reduce the risk of developing breast cancer by forty percent, I stopped using non-fat cow's milk and switched to non-fat soymilk.

My friends at The Wellness Community had also gotten the word on soy. Tina Rollo gave us her recipe for making soy shakes, and these became my favorite lunch. I take one-fourth to one-third of a package of firm, low-fat tofu and blend it with chocolate-flavored rice milk or soymilk. Of course the variations on this are endless just as adding a few ice cubes to the mix in the blender produces a thicker, icier shake. Tina liked to make her shake with tofu, ice, and orange juice. Others blended a package of frozen strawberries and a ripe banana with the tofu, making a thick fruit smoothie.

Before and after meetings we discussed the latest findings of this sort, and very often our interest in something like the soy craze would carry over into our support group discussions. We were always eager to share the latest, and we were overjoyed that finally—after too many years of ignoring most nutritional connections—researchers were looking into foods, vitamins, and herbal combinations that might enhance the body's ability to prevent cancer.

This is not to say, of course, that nutrition alone can prevent or cure cancer. Even if the cancer has not yet spread, and no conventional treatment (chemotherapy, surgery, radiation, etc.) is received, nutritional changes by themselves might not be enough. Researchers are claiming, however, that attention to what we eat can help the body's own immune system fight cancer cells while it also supports and restores healthy cells shot down by chemotherapy. The belief is that combining good nutrition with traditional treatment can boost the patient's chance for a cure. Nutritional imbalances in the body may weaken our immune systems to the point that a full-blown cancer can grow from a single cancerous cell that would ordinarily be sloughed off by the body's immune system.

But where do we begin? The claims are extensive. Cruciferous vegetables such as broccoli, cauliflower, bok choy, cabbage, and Brussels sprouts are alleged to have cancer-inhibiting substances that stop certain carcinogens before they have a chance to alter the DNA in a cancer cell thereby causing it to multiply out of control. I could easily live my whole life without cauliflower, but I forced myself to eat the others.

The so-called antioxidant vegetables (those high in vitamin A and beta-carotene) are among my favorites, so I don't have any trouble eating yams, sweet potatoes, carrots, spinach, asparagus, or raw bell peppers. Foods containing antioxidants are necessary to protect us against free radicals floating unchecked in the body.

Free radicals are molecules defined as having a single unpaired electron. These unfriendly little molecules can stimulate the division of mutated cells, kicking off a destructive chain reaction in the body. In addition to initiating various diseases, especially cancer, free radicals can also damage healthy cells. The solution to this free radical dilemma, we are told, is to stop the rampage of these toxic molecules and prevent disease with antioxidants such as vitamins A, C, and E and elements such as selenium.

After I read Dr. Andrew Weil's book, <u>Spontaneous Healing</u>, I began taking my vitamins and supplements according to his advice. I take 400 IU of vitamin E and 100 mcg of selenium at the same time (with breakfast) because they facilitate each other's absorption. But vitamin C can inhibit the absorption of selenium, so I take 500 mg of vitamin C later in the day (with my dinner).

Researchers at Tufts University in Boston found that patients who doubled their fruit and vegetable intake raised the antioxidant capability of their blood by thirteen to fifteen percent. Clearly the best way to improve antioxidant potential is through the foods we eat, but vitamin supplements that contain vitamins A, E, and C plus bioflavonoids, beta-carotene and selenium can also be effective cancer preventatives.

Research has shown that people with a high level of selenium in their blood, for example, have a lower incidence of cancer, but you have to be careful not to go hog-wild and swallow excessive doses of anything in pill form.

Green tea is also being recommended as a cancer preventative, possibly showing the same promise as soy. All teas, but especially green tea, contain powerful antioxidants called polyphenols. Studies claim that green tea is 100 times better than vitamin C as an antioxidant and 25 times more potent than vitamin E. The presence of Polyphenols in the body seems to decrease incidences of many cancers as well as protecting healthy cells from damage in cases of disease. Naturally this news sent everyone in my support group out in search of green tea.

Blandette Bush, Tina Rollo, and I attended several lectures on nutrition especially for cancer patients at The Wellness Community and ABC. Some doctors remain skeptical, but many are coming around to believe that diet and nutritional supplements can make a difference. We were taught that it is important for women with breast cancer to avoid meat or poultry that has been fed hormones because breast cancer (such as in my own case) can be hormone dependent.

We also learned that aside from the isoflavones in soy purportedly preventing the growth of some cancerous cells, the consumption of soy products might also lower the risk of osteoporosis, heart disease, and hot flashes. These problems become a real plague to those who've had breast or ovarian cancer because estrogen replacement hormones are not an option for them. Since I'm in this category, I try to eat soy every day not only to protect against more breast cancer, but also to reduce the torment of hot flashes. Oil of Evening Primrose is another supplement that I take daily because it is frequently recommended to help alleviate hot flashes. Oil of

Evening Primrose can be purchased in soft-gel capsules at most health food stores.

We were told to avoid fried foods, all animal dairy products, red meat, sugar, alcohol, coffee, and chocolate, but we could have all the soy, green tea, seaweed, and brown rice we wanted. It was sometimes hard to make healthy choices while maintaining a sense that we were not being sent to a dietary hell just because we'd had cancer.

It didn't take me long at all to get used to substituting soy protein for a good deal of the animal protein in my diet. I buy organic fruits and vegetables whenever I can, and Morrie has planted fruit trees in our yard to supply us with summer fruit that hasn't been sprayed with pesticides. I avoid strawberries altogether because of the pesticide problem and the difficulty in "scrubbing" a strawberry to remove any residue of pesticides.

I've met a few cancer patients who've gone all the way and switched to a totally macrobiotic diet. Macrobiotic nutrition involves attentive preparation of certain foods that are promoted as having special properties for fighting cancer. The regimen consists of carefully regulated daily portions of whole grains such as brown rice, leafy greens, round root vegetables, beans, nuts, seeds and seaweed.

Some cancer sufferers believe that a macrobiotic diet provides the reassurance that they are "doing" something positive by focusing on helping the body to restore its own immune system. I didn't have the energy to complete a rigorous changeover to macrobiotic cooking, but while researching the topic, I did come across some interesting recipes in Basic Macrobiotic Cooking by Julia Ferre.

Oriental doctors recommend this approach because they have always believed that paying attention to the daily diet is the most sensible way to approach any medical concern. The problem is, as I see it, that all too often a person will turn to something like a macrobiotic diet after they've reached an advanced stage of cancer and all else has failed. They've reached a point where the cancer has taken over completely and the immune system can no longer be strengthened by something as simple as a sweet potato or brown rice.

My own sense of logic tells me that I should have taken better care of myself starting many years ago. I couldn't go back and undo the fact that I ate a lot of junk in my youth, so I stopped eating it now. I eat lots of fruit and vegetables, and I make certain I drink plenty of water. I alternate between scrambled egg whites for breakfast (protein) and a high fiber cereal. I'm not strictly a vegetarian, but I do avoid red meat because of the fear of added hormones. I get most of my protein from soy, fish, and hormone-free chicken. I eliminated butter, vegetable oils, and margarine from my diet, and I now use extra-virgin olive oil as my main source of fat.

Since many breast cancer victims are overweight, some believe the fat theory still deserves close scrutiny, but there's a catch to that approach as well. I read The Zone by Dr. Barry Sears and learned that you have to eat a certain amount of fat in order to lose fat. He explains how the fat-free craze has actually "fattened" the American people. Many people who've gone on the fashionable low fat, high-carbohydrate diets are actually putting themselves in dietary danger, all the while thinking they are doing the "right" thing.

I also went to a homeopath and got some advice regarding herbs and homeopathic remedies. I cleared all this with Dr. Chang, of course, and I continue to take herbal dietary supplements, again to bolster my immune system. Since the liver has to process all the substances that enter the bloodstream, when I take my prescribed Tamoxifen tablets, for example, I also take a capsule of milk thistle extract, a supplement that supports normal liver function.

On the down side, the growing demand for herbs and other supplements holds a certain risk for the consumer. These products are not tested or regulated nearly as closely as over-the-counter drugs or even foods. Questionable herbal preparations have been found to contain toxic levels of mercury, arsenic, lead, and other heavy metals. The consumer should not equate the word "natural" with safe or wholesome. Arsenic and many other deadly substances are found "naturally" in the environment.

Just about everyone in my group at The Wellness Community has tried one dietary fad or another. Some tried something new every week. We were always tempted to latch onto a newly recommended remedy, even if it meant drinking six cups of a terrible-tasting tea every day or enduring a coffee enema. While many believed they were going for a "cure," most of us realized that alternative therapies were not intended to destroy cancer, but rather to reduce symptoms while strengthening our own immune systems.

If we heard or read about someone being cured of cancer simply because she'd thrown away all her aluminum pots and pans, the next logical step was for us to go home and do likewise. I couldn't follow up on that advice, however, because I'd already thrown away all my aluminum pots at least ten years earlier after reading a claim that cooking in aluminum could possibly cause Alzheimers Disease.

By discussing the latest "cures" for cancer, we learned to investigate the scientific basis for a claim before we ingested something that might be questionable. Sometimes adding a strange new food or supplement to our diet actually created stress and more stress was definitely one thing we didn't need. In other words, the cancer patient should try anything and everything that might help, but good sense should always be a part of the equation.

Fallen Soldiers

I wasn't exactly sad to see 1996 come to an end. January of 1997 marked my one-year anniversary since the mastectomy. It's almost universal that cancer survivors celebrate milestones of their recovery more zealously than birthdays and anniversaries of events that took place B. C. (before cancer). I was also overjoyed that I'd lived to see the birth of our first grandson, Ryan Christopher Rosen, born to Scott and Ellen on April 4, 1997. We now had five beautiful grandchildren.

My hair continued to grow, coming in silver and very curly, quite different from the straight brown hair I'd had before. It was a whole new look for me—hair so short there was no way to style it that didn't give me the appearance of a punk rocker. Young sales clerks in stores would notice, complimenting me on my great "haircut" and the hair "color" I'd selected. The younger they were, the more excited they would become over my daring attempt to be a part of their more enlightened generation. Cancer was obviously not a part of their daily experience, and I didn't have the heart to tell sixteen-year-olds about the horrors of chemotherapy. Better they should think I was some sort of really cool grandma.

At the end of April, I reached another anniversary, one year since my surgery for the ovarian cancer. A few weeks later, Sharron Goldstein lost her struggle with ovarian cancer. She had been treated for gastritis for many months before her problem was accurately diagnosed, a tragic refrain I'd heard far too many times. It didn't feel right celebrating my own survival when others in my support group had lost the battle. I couldn't help feeling guilty that I was one of the lucky ones.

I was okay, I kept telling myself. I was cured, cancer-free, in remission, whatever. Then a woman came to The Wellness Community who had undergone a mastectomy the previous year, about the same time as I had. Our cases seemed to be identical. Her lymph nodes had shown no evidence of cancer, so her prognosis was, like mine, very encouraging. Also like me, her doctor had placed her on Tamoxifen.

She assumed that her battle with breast cancer had been won, but then she went on to explain to the group that she'd been having back pain. The pain became severe, so the tests began. A bone biopsy finally revealed metastatic breast cancer in her spine.

I was shocked. If it had happened to her, it could also happen to me, but I never voiced this fear to her. In fact, I never uttered a negative word about anything in her presence. We all emphasized that at The Wellness Community we made it a rule never to think that our lives were over, as long as there was hope, no matter how slim. One of the first things I'd learned at The Wellness Community was that as long as a person is alive, there is hope.

But the poor woman was depressed; she believed her life was over. We all tried to tell her that this kind of thinking was not productive, that negative thought or activity actually drains the energy or life force from cell tissue. For many years medical researchers have been aware that negative emotions caused negative chemical reactions in the body. And now scientists are even acknowledging that positive emotions can also generate a change. It appears likely that depression and despair certainly might hinder the body's ability to heal.

But members of the group also learned how to face the inevitable when the time came. Only when all treatment options were exhausted, and our positive thinking had done all it could possibly do, then and only then would it be okay to shift our thinking to embrace the inner peace associated with accepting death. At the very end, when the cancer gained final control, our mutual goal would be to pray for strength to derive joy from the days we had left.

Unfortunately, she wasn't buying any of it, and within a month she died. In 1997 we also lost Jackie Watt to esophageal cancer and Lloyd Isham to a brain tumor.

Whenever a member of our support group passed away, we all grieved. Except for those who were going through the worst days of chemotherapy, we always attended funerals and memorial services together, and we cried together. By the same token, with each goodbye we learned. We learned how fleeting life actually is, and we learned to appreciate every minute of every day. Somehow our grief made us strong.

Following a death, we would come together, feeling anger at cancer in general. This open anger helped us to vent some of our frustrations, so in that sense the anger wasn't a bad emotion. Anger was, in fact, a powerful catalyst that made us want to fight even harder to overcome our own cancers.

We would always devote at least part of our weekly meeting to our most recently fallen soldier. We talked about death and our anger because we'd lost a friend. No one held back. Our true feelings just poured out, and in the process, the unexpected frequently popped up.

It was at these most intense times in our group that one of us would realize that he or she needed to come to terms with a spouse, child, or parent in order to settle some old business. The need to make amends with family and friends seemed to be a natural offshoot of our newly acquired (positive) thinking.

Sometimes these feelings surfaced more or less out of the blue, and frequently our discussions spawned an overdue reconciliation with a loved one. Making peace with an estranged family member was considered necessary to some, but many times the opposite occurred. Occasionally a decision to sever all ties with a relative came out during one of these reflective sessions. We often heard tales of a relative or even a friend who was dragging down the cancer patient by acting entirely too selfish or insensitive. We all agreed it was a good idea to avoid pessimists no matter what the family connection might be.

At these times my civilian friends would again wonder why I would knowingly become so close to someone who had little chance of survival. For my initial response I would simply state that a support group was not about giving in to cancer. Hope was always an important part of our belief system. We further maintained that a diagnosis of cancer is not an automatic death sentence. By fighting and holding on to our beliefs, our strength grew.

Secondly, there was no way we could walk away from our friends who were having a hard time. Those participants who couldn't handle the group dynamics didn't stay with the group for very long. Cancer survivors within a support group don't treat each other as someone doomed to die, even though the topic of death comes up frequently. Cancer survivors in a support group become friends, very close friends.

By the fall of 1997, Maria Alvarez was running out of options. She was back on chemotherapy, and she was also receiving radiation treatments for the larger, more painful tumors in her bones. She'd heard about a clinical trial that was being conducted at UCLA for women with advanced cases of breast or ovarian cancer and asked her doctor to look into it. Early reports claimed that one woman in the trial had gone into complete remission of advanced metastatic breast cancer and others had reported drastic reductions in tumor size.

Dr. Dennis Slamon, Chief of the Division of Hematology and Oncology and Executive Vice Chair for Research within the Department of Medicine at UCLA, was in charge of this clinical trial. The study involved women whose tumors had turned especially aggressive due to over-production of a protein generated by a gene called HER-2/neu within the cancer cell itself. This protein appeared to regulate the growth of the tumor.

The drug they were testing was manufactured by Genentech in South San Francisco and was later named Herceptin. This genetically engineered antibody adheres to the HER-2/neu receptor and inhibits the cancer's growth. On the down side, however, only about thirty-percent of all breast and ovarian cancer tumors respond to this new treatment because the protein (from the HER-2/neu receptor) has to be present in the cancer cells for the antibody to do its work.

Maria was not only in that slim thirty-percent category, but according to her oncologist also at UCLA, she was a perfect candidate to receive help from this drug. We were euphoric! We prayed. We shouted.

Maria could be on her way to a complete recovery.

Maria

As little as ten to fifteen years ago research into genetic engineering to develop a cure for breast cancer was still young. No one believed mammalian cells (cells from a mammal) could be manufactured. Almost accidentally, back in 1986, Dr. Dennis Slamon of UCLA and ex-Genentech researcher Alex Ulrich discovered that a protein produced by the HER-2/neu gene is over-expressed in about twenty to thirty percent of breast cancers. They believed this protein was responsible for cell growth so research continued. They further reasoned that an antibody could be developed to shut down cancer cell "signals" for the cell to grow and divide. The antibody had to be "humanized" so mammalian cells (taken from hamsters) were used to manufacture the drug, and by 1991 the development of Herceptin was under way.

Although it was not claimed to be a miracle drug, Herceptin had exhibited some miraculous results in some patients and Maria was excited. Clinical trials of Herceptin had been on going for several years and the third and final phase of the testing had begun in April of 1995. Over seven hundred women at one hundred different testing sites had received this highly experimental drug as part of the study. Since it was too late for Maria to actually enter the trial, her doctor submitted a request for the drug to be administered to her for compassionate reasons.

The problem was that the drug was being manufactured in very limited quantities. It had not yet received FDA approval, so the company was allowed to produce only the amount needed for the trials plus a small additional allotment that was intended for desperately ill patients, like Maria, on a strictly compassionate basis. In order to assure that this apportioning would be fair to all women who were in need, the National Breast Cancer Coalition requested distribution by a computerized lottery system. Since the NBCC had already been instrumental in overseeing patient safety in these trials, their input was accepted.

So Maria's name went into a computerized hat. The first lottery rolled around, but Maria's name was not selected. She was disappointed, of course, but we tried to talk about other things to get her mind off the HER-2/neu lottery.

More often than not, Maria wanted to discuss her daughter Jennifer's up-coming wedding. The wedding had originally been scheduled for June 1998, but in light of her mother's illness, Jennifer had moved the date up to December 1997. Maria was determined to attend her daughter's wedding and not even her ever-increasing bone pain could discourage her. Her doctor gave her a morphine pump to supply her with a steady flow of pain medication, but she was still thinking positively. Cancer may have attacked Maria's body but not her spirit.

Three weeks later another lottery was held; Maria did not win. Maria and I scheduled a date to go out for lunch, but when the day arrived, she was feeling much too tired to go anywhere. In fact right about this time she was also forced to stop attending our support group at The Wellness Community for the same reason. We all kept in touch with her by phone. She was always delighted when I called, but her voice sounded unsteady and so very fragile.

Maria missed having her name come up again in November and by now we'd learned that her breast cancer had invaded her brain. The lottery process of making certain an experimental drug was distributed fairly suddenly seemed contemptible and senseless. We didn't want to hear that the drug couldn't be distributed without fear of reprisal until it had received full FDA approval. We didn't care about federal red tape.

We wrote letters to UCLA and Genentech, attempting to let the people in charge know that Maria did not have a whole lot of time left. They were sympathetic but they had no choice other than continuing to distribute the precious few available doses of Herceptin via the lottery. When our group met at The Wellness Community we shouted in anger, feeling helpless and very much afraid for Maria.

Finally, after losing the lottery so many times, Maria's name was selected by the computer. The drug was given to her at once, but even Maria knew that it was too late. She had grown much weaker and was now unable to leave her bed. She was drained from all the treatments and drugs and the endless visits to UCLA, and of course the pain from the growing tumors in her bones was sapping her strength.

Her daughter Jennifer's wedding date was rapidly approaching, but the family was concerned that Maria might not last even a few more days. A priest was summoned to their home, and he married Jennifer and Sean in Maria's bedroom.

I went to see Maria a few days later, and as frail as she was, she was still talking about attending her daughter's church wedding before she died. Death was etched on her face. I choked up, and I couldn't prevent a few tears from spilling down my cheeks.

Maria said, "It's all right, Marion. I just want to be there for Jennifer's wedding, and then I'll be ready."

As I left Maria's house and walked across the tree-lined street to my car, I began to sob. I sat alone in my car for a long while, crying and feeling certain that I'd never see Maria again. But I was forgetting the moral strength of this extraordinary woman. It took some time for me to digest all that I was learning from Maria.

A week later Maria attended her daughter's wedding. She was in a wheelchair, but she was there. Maria's husband, David, drove her home to rest after the church service, but then, later in the day, he took her to the wedding reception for a brief appearance.

Maria celebrated Christmas with her family, and over the holidays Amelia Prince, from our support group, and I went to visit her. Amelia had been a scrub nurse, working for many years in the operating rooms at a nearby Veterans Administration Hospital.

Expecting to see a dying woman, we were overjoyed to find Maria sitting up in bed, fully dressed and wearing her favorite hat and earrings. She had even applied lipstick and a faint layer of makeup. She showed us the dress and matching hat she'd worn to Jennifer's wedding, and she bragged non-stop about how handsome her son John had looked in his tuxedo. She was animated, excited actually, as she told us all about the wonderful feelings of love and exhilaration she'd experienced at her daughter's wedding. She had danced at her daughter's wedding, if only in her heart, and her spirit had soared to an incredible high.

It was a wonderful visit with the three of us sprawled on Maria's king size bed like teenagers at a slumber party. We laughed a lot. We cried a little. Maria asked dozens of questions about the other members of our support group. She wanted to hear about events that Amelia and I had planned with our families. I told her all about our itinerary for an Alaskan cruise and land trip that we'd scheduled for the following July. Maria wanted to know every detail regarding Amelia's plans for a combined camping trip and family reunion.

Maria wanted to go with David to see the same sights that we were planning to see. She wanted to hear about fun and families. She wanted to see our photographs. She savored anecdotes about the latest escapades of my five grandchildren, good times with grandchildren that Maria would never know.

We all must die, but the secret is to do it with the kind of dignity that flowed so naturally from Maria. If one must die, do it well.

Maria passed away on January 7, 1998.

Herceptin was the first biologic therapy approved by the FDA for the treatment of cancer. It was given FDA approval in September of 1998, and mass distribution to the medical community was immediately launched ten days later. Approval was won too late to save Maria, but it is encouraging to know that many others will have their disease slowed or even completely reversed by this radically new drug.

Death is a part of life. Facing Maria's death along with her taught me a lot about life, and I now appreciate how unpredictable a hold we have on it. This gossamer thing we call life seems too precarious by far for mere humans to comprehend.

I had survived four major surgeries and some industrial-strength chemotherapy, but my friend had died. We assume all too readily that those we love will always be with us. We learn they won't.

I remember Maria's courage, and I am grateful that I was blessed with her love. Maria taught me that it is essential that I should enhance my life in whatever way that is important to me alone.

My longtime friend Pat Klein from northern California (and also a breast cancer survivor) had been in constant contact by phone, listening to my cancer tale as it unfolded. She sent me many "love" gifts, one a verse printed in lovely calligraphy. The author was not identified, but it stated the feelings in my heart so poignantly that I had it reproduced on a heavy cardstock paper. I made enough copies to give one to each person in my support group. It goes like this:

Cancer might rob you of that blissful ignorance that once led you to believe that tomorrow stretched forever.

In exchange you are granted the vision of seeing each day as a precious gift to be used richly and wisely.

When you accept these words and live by them, each day really does become precious.

Cancer, Cancer Everywhere

Losing Maria was hard on all of us. She had fought so valiantly, yet her cancer just couldn't be arrested. We worked through our grief together during our support group, but we all felt the pain. The reality of cancer was harsh and exacting, and it never seemed to relent.

Meanwhile, outside of my group at The Wellness Community, cancer, especially breast cancer, was cropping up within our family and circle of friends. My sister-in-law, Carol Rosen, the most thoughtful woman I've ever known, had a bout with breast cancer.

Our daughter Deborah's mother-in-law, Jean Kiel, had to undergo surgery for colon cancer.

Then my close friend Nancy Fisher was diagnosed with breast cancer. I wished I could be with her as she underwent surgery and then radiation, but Nancy had recently moved from California to Washington, DC. Her husband Ray Fisher had received a presidential appointment to serve as Associate Attorney General of the United States, which was, of course, a very prestigious position. I kept assuring myself that Washington had wonderful doctors while I continued to worry about Nancy.

Just a few weeks later, my friend Peggy Stabile, a high school counselor, was diagnosed with breast cancer. Naturally Peggy was frightened. I spoke to her frequently and encouraged her to transfer from her Kaiser facility to mine so she could request Dr. Schilling and Dr. Chang. She made the change and was pleased with the physicians I'd recommended, but Peggy also learned that facing breast cancer is never easy.

While Peggy was still undergoing treatment, another dear friend, Felice Anspacher, told me she'd found a lump in her breast. Felice's husband Lee taught history at the same high school where I'd taught, and Morrie and I had shared many wonderful evenings with these two steadfast, marvelous friends. The four of us always cracked jokes and laughed the whole time we were together. With Felice's diagnosis of breast cancer, suddenly we were no longer laughing.

Next, my friend in New York, Bettina Ling, called to tell me her mother, Betty Ling, had breast cancer.

Another longtime friend, Judy Heckman, told me her darling mother Grace Hinnershitz, who I'd known since childhood, was diagnosed with a rare optic cancer.

Our friend Marge Brinkworth from Pennsylvania had extensive surgery and bladder reconstruction for bladder cancer.

David Baker, Ruth and Allen's son, had a melanoma removed from his chest.

Gerry Poeschel, a friend who was also the realtor who had found our current house for us, discovered she had uterine cancer.

It seemed that every time the phone rang, I received news about yet another diagnosis of cancer. How could so many people I cared about have cancer? Seeing these good people suffering from such insidious cancers was enough to make me want to scream.

I was now exercising at the YMCA, trying to stay fit by attending water aerobics classes. Almost every woman in our class was aware that I had lost a breast to cancer. Showering and changing in front of many other women made it difficult to keep something like that a secret. One day in the locker room a young woman named Molly approached me. She explained that she had discovered a lump in her breast and she was obviously worried. She asked me to take a look at it.

At first I hesitated. I had absolutely no medical training, and I certainly had no business examining another woman's lump. I was about to tell her to see a doctor, but then I spotted the fear in Molly's eyes. I knew how it felt to be on the verge of shattering like glass. She needed a friend, preferably one who had survived breast cancer, and she needed that friend on the spot.

Molly directed my finger to a rather large lump on the lower outer quadrant of her right breast. Suddenly I was worried, too. I echoed the words I had heard so often and gently explained that it was probably nothing more than a harmless cyst. Even as I reassured her, I made it very clear that she needed to see a doctor at once.

Fortunately, Molly took my advice without hesitation and went directly to her doctor. The lump turned out to be a benign cyst, and when she reported her good news, everyone in the women's locker room cheered. I was delighted that this was one round cancer had lost.

My visits to Dr. Chang's office every three months served to further remind me that cancer was everywhere. With so many people making return appointments to the same department, I began to recognize folks I'd seen in the oncology waiting room previously. Some of my friends from The Wellness Community went to the same Kaiser Medical Center, so I would run into them, also. There was always a sad kind of camaraderie in that waiting room, a feeling that we were all in this together, as people discreetly inquired about one another's health. Aside from changing one's life entirely, cancer gives even total strangers this connection, an unspoken kinship, however temporary.

I was still receiving the tumor marker tests on a regular basis. I'd just had the CA 2729 for breast cancer and the CA 125 for ovarian cancer. This time my CA 2729 reading had been slightly elevated, but fluctuation in test scores is usually not a major cause for alarm. The tests have a normal margin of error, but in spite of the fact that they are not foolproof, they are still probably the best hope for early detection of a recurrence.

It had been more than a year since my last full-body CT scan so, in light of my elevated tumor marker reading, Dr. Chang ordered another. I went for the scan February 3, 1998, and Dr. Chang called me shortly thereafter. He reported that the radiologist had detected a 3mm. nodule along the periphery of my left lower lung. It was located in such a place that a needle biopsy could not be performed safely. He recommended that we wait a month and then do another scan to see whether the nodule had grown. If so, Dr. Chang recommended that I should have the open chest surgery that would be required to biopsy the spot. He also mentioned that ninety percent of metastatic breast cancer spreads to the lungs, liver, or bones.

Deja vu. Another surgery? Open chest surgery—which is always risky—just to perform a biopsy? Although the fear of recurrence is a persistent annoyance that lurks somewhere in the back of every cancer survivor's mind, I had psyched myself into believing that I was one of the lucky ones. If I was so lucky, why did I suddenly have a spot in my lung?

I'd already tried chemotherapy, so this time I tried shopping therapy. I went on an offensive attack at the mall. I bought new clothes and frivolous things for the house. I found a plump new designer comforter for our bed and matching sheets to go with it. I planned a counterattack at the shoe store and bought four new pairs of dressy shoes that I didn't need. Heck, I didn't need even one pair.

Once the shopping therapy had run its course, I telephoned my friend Gertrude Pomish and she convinced me that I needed to see a pulmonary specialist, a man she trusted and respected because he'd treated a friend of hers for many years. Gertrude arranged an appointment for me with Dr. Martin Gordon in Beverly Hills.

I went to Kaiser and checked out all the film from my most recent CT scan as well as the film from the previous one. A full CT scan involves about ninety-six pictures, so Morrie had a heavy load to carry the day we went to see Dr. Gordon.

Dr. Gordon chatted with us briefly and then began scrutinizing my CT scans, especially the previous one. It didn't take him long to identify the very same nodule on the earlier scan. It had been there well over a year, and it hadn't grown at all. The Kaiser radiologist had obviously missed it the first time around because he'd been so busy focusing on the large cystic mass in my pelvis that later turned out to be the ovarian cancer. The spot has never been identified for certain, but Dr. Chang and Dr. Gordon both suspected it was scar tissue that resulted from an attack of pneumonia I'd had twenty years earlier.

I didn't know whether to laugh or cry. I had a feeling these brief skirmishes with the fear of recurring cancer would somehow become a part of my life from now on.

Bonus Time

Right about the time I was dealing with the spot in my lung, Barbara Foerster and her husband Roy went on a mineral collecting expedition, a passion they had enjoyed together for years. The high point of this trip was a visit to the "Cave of Swords" in northeastern Mexico, one of the foremost wonders of the mineralogical world. Since it is closed to the public, they had to obtain special permission to enter this extraordinary cave. The walls are covered with protruding selenite crystals ranging from a few inches to several feet in length, the larger ones truly looking like colossal swords of crystal being wielded by some unseen giant.

A trip of this nature would've been nearly impossible for anyone else with an advanced stage of cancer, but Barbara was up for it. She may have been tired and short of breath while they explored the depths of this spectacular cavern, but she savored every minute. She wore a hard hat with its own beacon of light as she and Roy followed their personal guide down many feet below the surface of the Earth.

Before Barbara left on this adventure she'd been advised that her chemotherapy was no longer working. Just as strains of bacteria somehow learn to resist certain antibiotics, cancer cells can become resistant to the chemicals being used to treat it. Chemotherapy doesn't always kill cancer completely, but it does usually shrink tumors and help the patient to live longer. Barb's ovarian cancer was spreading, and she knew that she would soon reach the point when she would have to make some serious decisions about continuing treatment.

Barbara also knew that I had been faced with this very same dilemma, and we talked about it. She praised me for taking control of my treatment, but I cautioned her that my prognosis had been quite different from hers. Barbara's cancer had spread extensively before it had even been diagnosed, so although more than three years of constant chemotherapy had kept the cancer at bay, it was still there. A recent CT scan had showed tumor growth in her right lung, on the chest wall, and throughout her abdominal cavity.

The day after their return from Mexico, Barbara sought additional advice from a top gynecological oncologist at Cedars Sinai Hospital in Beverly Hills. She had a brief glimmer of hope that more surgery might be viable, but in the end all her doctors agreed the cancer was too widespread to even consider surgery. Barbara was scheduled to begin another series of chemical infusions with a brand new drug that had just been approved by the FDA in January 1998, but she was wise enough to realize that it was time to reconcile to the inevitable.

Barbara had fought a long, hard battle, but like Maria, she had grown weary of the debilitating side effects of chemotherapy. She decided she would terminate all chemotherapy treatment. But giving up treatment is not the same as giving up.

Barb knew her cancer could not be cured, but she was not fearful. She spoke of death calmly and courageously because her absolute faith in God gave her tremendous comfort.

She said, "I'm now in the hands of the Lord, and the Lord will give me the strength to face whatever comes in the months ahead."

Barbara and Roy were determined to enjoy however many days she had left rather than dwell on the fact that the cancer was in full control. Barbara remained in good spirits even though her strength was rapidly diminishing. During the summer of 1998, she continued to attend our support group at The Wellness Community and she never missed church on Sundays. By now she was enjoying these and other activities in a wheelchair, but she saw the wheelchair simply as an expedient way to get where she wanted to go.

She treasured each new day as a supreme gift—still using the term bonus time—and she always focused on the day that stretched before her rather than the time that would never be. Every minute of life was so precious to Barbara that she refused to waste a single moment on self-pity or negative thoughts.

Even after Barbara's chemotherapy had lost its ability to hold her disease at bay, her will to live kept her going for many more months than anyone (including her doctors) would have believed possible. We said she was like the "Energizer" pink bunny because she miraculously just kept going.

She knew she had to live her life to the fullest in case tomorrow didn't come, and live it she did. She was even thankful her situation had given her plenty of time to say goodbye to her loved ones. There was never any mention of how much time she might have left, only how that time could be spent.

For Barb, survival was not geared to a definitive period of weeks or months but rather to making it through one day at a time, and she greeted each glorious day with an enormous supply of courage. Psalm 118:24 truly echoed her motto: "This is the day which the Lord has made; we will rejoice and be glad in it."

Much of her time was spent giving compassionate, supportive love to others with cancer. Whenever someone at The Wellness Community lashed out at God or at the world in general, angry because they had cancer, it was always Barbara who reined them in with her gentle, loving way. She provided sympathetic attention, invariably comforting others with her unbelievable strength. Her willingness to be there for the rest of us was downright amazing. Here was a woman who could have spent her final days in self-pity, but instead she concentrated on helping others.

Because of Barbara I have also learned that love must be a very positive enhancement of the body's immune system. Love kept her going, and in turn, we were all convinced that the most important thing in life is love. The second most important thing is sharing that love.

From Snake Oil to Shark Cartilage

As long as people are afflicted with dreadful diseases like cancer, proponents of unconventional treatments will abound. The fast-talking snake oil peddlers who preyed on our ancestors look a bit different nowadays, but the greediness of charlatans who want to strike it rich at the expense of someone who is critically ill probably will never disappear.

Of course there are many treatments for cancer that are promoted by honest individuals who would truly like to rid the world of this disease. Complementary or alternative medicine usually focuses on helping the body to restore its own immune system or to eliminate toxins through things like diet, vitamins, herbal or medicinal supplements, and teas, all the while strengthening the belief that the state of the mind and body are linked. Some herbal preparations, for example, can help the patient cope with pain and stress. With pain and stress under control, the patient is more likely to be able to tolerate further traditional (and toxic) forms of treatment such as chemotherapy.

Many alternative treatments offer no anti-cancer benefits that have ever been recognized in scientific circles, but patients still swear they are being helped. Of course, if you also consider hope and the patient's own belief system, we know that even a placebo can work miracles. The American Cancer Society and the National Cancer Institute urge patients to seek a doctor's advice before <u>combining</u> high doses of herbal formulas or antioxidants with chemotherapy, however. Extremely high amounts of some antioxidants can interfere with conventional chemicals to the point that the benefits of the chemotherapy are neutralized.

Regardless of the source of unproven cancer therapies, it is wise to do a little research before investing money in something that may present unknown risks to the patient. Literally hundreds of cancer remedies that are not considered to be scientifically effective have surfaced in the last fifty years, and it is estimated that Americans spend $500 million annually on unorthodox cancer treatments. I even came across a web site that provides information to help cancer patients examine and sift through the claims. www.quackwatch.com

The best example of an unproven cancer remedy is probably Laetrile. I checked www.quackwatch.com and discovered dozens of papers and articles describing this substance and its connection with cancer. The American Cancer Society has contributed a lengthy article to the Internet titled <u>Laetrile Background Information</u>. Dr. Benjamin Wilson also provides factual information in his commentary, <u>The Rise and Fall of Laetrile</u>.

Laetrile is the trade name for laevo-mandelonitrile-beta-glucuronoside, patented by Ernst T. Krebs, Jr. in 1952. In the 1920's, Krebs's father, Dr. Ernst T. Krebs, Sr. tested an extract of apricot kernels that contained amygdalin. (The word amygdalin is often used interchangeably with Laetrile.)

The senior Krebs found Laetrile too toxic for medicinal purposes because amygdalin breaks down into hydrogen cyanide, a deadly poison. Years later, Krebs Jr., who had no medical training, claimed he had refined his father's formula, and he began to manufacture and distribute Laetrile as a cure for cancer.

For more than twenty years, various scientific studies concluded that Laetrile did not cause tumors to shrink, nor did it increase the patient's survival time. In spite of its embattled history, Laetrile has been pursued by legions of desperate cancer patients who have gone to incredible lengths to receive treatments. No one can truly understand how frenzied people can become following a diagnosis of cancer unless they've been there themselves. Some patients actually died of cyanide poisoning after taking Laetrile, and many others might have been saved if they'd accepted appropriate conventional chemotherapy instead of gambling on Laetrile. Unfortunately it is always hard to convince distressed patients of these findings.

Many swore by Laetrile as it slowly poisoned them, claiming "conspiracy charges" against those in the U.S. government who attempted to ban the substance. The legal battles over Laetrile eventually made it all the way to the United States Supreme Court. The Supreme Court's 1979 ruling declared it illegal to transport Laetrile across state lines or from another country into the U.S., even with a physician's affidavit. Before Congress, Senator Edward Kennedy openly criticized Laetrile backers as "slick salesmen who would offer a false sense of hope" to cancer patients.

One American woman found a doctor in Mexico who was willing to administer Laetrile injections to her. The woman became convinced that Laetrile had saved her life, and the word spread rapidly. She eventually died of her cancer, but during the years she lived in remission, she actively promoted the drug, and hundreds flocked across the California border into Mexico to receive Laetrile. As a result of this fanatic search for a cure for cancer, Dr. Ernesto Contreras had earned enough to expand his tiny Mexican clinic into a large, modern hospital.

In 1980, actor Steve McQueen praised his treatment with Laetrile, and this further publicity sent more Americans across the border. Steve McQueen died shortly after his Laetrile treatments in Mexico, but his endorsement alone was enough to encourage other cancer patients to give it a try.

Several additional cancer treatment centers opened in Mexico just south of the California line, and many are still operating today. Patients stay in comfortable motels on the California side of the border and travel back and forth for treatment.

In short, no measurable benefit from Laetrile has ever been recorded, but even to this day, Laetrile is available for purchase via the Internet. In spite of the law and the fact that the American Cancer Society strongly urges patients with cancer not to use Laetrile, some individuals still travel to distant locations and pay hefty prices for Laetrile treatments.

In some cases, the patient's unwavering belief in the treatment might be all that Laetrile can actually offer, but of course, we must not discount the fact that belief <u>alone</u> is a very powerful medicine.

In the spring of 1998, Tina Rollo, from my support group at The Wellness Community, found she was running out of treatment options. She had received high dose chemotherapy without a stem cell rescue following her second mastectomy, and as a result her bone marrow had shut down. This meant her bone marrow was not producing new white and red blood cells, and her blood counts were far too low for her to undergo additional chemotherapy.

Her doctors explored the possibility of a bone marrow transplant, but no suitable donor could be found in spite of the fact that she had five siblings. While the doctors patiently waited for her bone marrow to recover sufficiently to resume blood cell production on its own, Tina got busy on the Internet. She wasn't about to just sit back and wait. If there was anything that could be done to facilitate her way to recovery, Tina was determined to discover it. While surfing the web, trying to track down possibilities for clinical trials, she came across the results of a study that had been conducted by a grad student from China who was doing research at Emory University.

Twenty-nine-year-old Keqiang Ye had discovered that Noscapine, an ingredient found in common cough syrups, possessed the remarkable ability to stop tumor cells from dividing in laboratory mice, and then the Noscapine killed the cancer cells completely. This discovery had to be tested further via clinical trials since Noscapine had never received FDA approval in the U.S., but Tina learned that the cough suppressant had been available in Sweden, Japan, and South Africa for years. Tina made many telephone calls until she finally found someone in Sweden who was willing to mail her the cough syrup. She had no idea how much Noscapine

115

to take, so she took the maximum dosage recommended for a severe cold.

Tina also explored many other avenues of alternative care. She found a Chinese herbalist who gave her a bag of dried, ground herbs she was supposed to mix with water and brew into a murky-looking "tea." We jokingly called it her bag of dirt, but she drank the concoction religiously for some months. She also tried Essiac tea, another non-toxic herbal cancer remedy from Canada. Essiac is made from four common herbs and does not have FDA approval, but supporters maintain it shrinks tumors.

Neither homeopathy nor Chinese medicine actually makes a claim that its methods will cure cancer, but countless patients successfully use homeopathic or Chinese formulas to alleviate pain and to reduce nausea and other side effects of chemotherapy.

Many people who try herbal remedies to fight cancer are hoping to bolster their body's immune system, in order that the immune system itself can become strong enough to do the job of destroying the tumor. Some are hoping to circumvent surgery or chemotherapy altogether.

Tina had not gotten into alternative treatments because she wanted to avoid traditional chemotherapy or radiation. She would have been thrilled to zap her breast cancer with chemicals. She was exploring every possible alternative because, with her bone marrow not functioning, nothing else was available to her. She tried to bolster her immune system in every conceivable way.

Tina also experimented with shark cartilage to battle her cancer. The publication of <u>Sharks Don't Get Cancer</u> by I. William Lane, Ph.D. and Linda Comac in 1992 set off a Laetrile-like commotion over preparations created from the cartilage of shark skeletons. Usually in capsule form, shark cartilage is sold in health food stores as a supplement rather than a drug and therefore does not require FDA approval.

Although the protein found in shark cartilage won't hurt, most researchers have insisted there is absolutely no clinical evidence that shark cartilage does anything more than hold a shark together. Undaunted, Dr. Lane came back with his second book on the subject, Sharks Still Don't Get Cancer, in 1996. A study reported in the Journal of Clinical Oncology in 1998 stated that shark cartilage supplements failed to slow the spread of cancer or even to improve the patient's quality of life. Nevertheless, Aeterna Labs is waiting approval on a new drug that contains shark cartilage. They hope to use this drug to destroy blood vessels in lung and prostate tumors.

Tina's bone marrow eventually kicked in and her blood counts slowly improved. She was placed on low dosage chemotherapy, but by this time there was evidence that her breast cancer had spread to her lungs. She continued on chemotherapy, but also sought acupuncture as a means of finding relief from the side effects of the chemotherapy. Acupuncture can also help relieve stress and anxiety for the cancer patient.

Tina devoted every waking moment to reinforcing her health-enhancing behavior. She didn't want her three daughters ages nine, eleven, and thirteen to see her as a crazed fanatic, so she made every effort to "normalize" her endless array of cancer therapies. She also made a point to avoid any show of fear around her daughters. Tina would have been the last one to say that her course of action was exceptional, but I always felt that she displayed an unparalleled amount of wisdom and courage.

Next, Tina found a clinical trial being conducted at a hospital in Nashville, Tennessee. The study was using a vaccine produced from live tumor cells in order to stimulate the patient's own defenses to establish a natural immunity against the cancer.

Tina was accepted into the trial, but of course she had to fly to Nashville on a regular basis to receive inoculations of the vaccine. Travel for trial participation usually has to be done at the patient's own expense, but Tina got busy on the phone and soon discovered that most U.S. commercial airlines will transport cancer patients to treatment centers across the country at greatly reduced rates.

In addition to the vaccine she was given in Nashville, Tina also received traditional chemotherapy at home to further diminish the number of cancer cells the vaccine had to fight.

It was summertime and school was out, so usually one of her three daughters went along with her to Nashville. In spite of her rapidly failing health, Tina lavished plenty of extra attention on the daughter who went along for the ride. Somehow Tina always managed to turn a wearisome therapeutic treatment into an exciting adventure for one of her girls.

Tina fought long and hard. She persevered with treatments in Nashville even as the level of cancer in her body continued to rise. Tina and many others I've met at The Wellness Community found both positives and negatives in their various alternative treatments. But Tina felt good about "doing" something to help herself, so we encouraged her to try anything and everything. Sadly, it still wasn't enough.

For many patients, however, refusing traditional medicine isn't a question of risk. When traditional chemotherapy ceases to provide any benefit for the patient, it doesn't make sense to suffer all the discomforts of chemotherapy's side effects. Barbara Foerster had reached that very same conclusion with her decision to quit chemotherapy

If the patient's prognosis isn't good, and chemotherapy cannot continue to extend life, it seems logical to find solace in an alternative treatment providing the cost of such treatment isn't exorbitant. Most alternative choices are considered experimental and are therefore not covered by insurance.

By taking control of treatment or by making other significant lifestyle changes, the patient has taken a step away from the frightening cycle of total dependency on his or her physician. As the last days of a cancer patient's life unfold, being the one in charge of any treatment, including an alternative one, can be a tremendous source of peace of mind.

Barbara's Last Hallelujah

By October 1998, Barbara Foerster had grown much weaker, and she was spending her days in bed or in a wheelchair. Her husband Roy had set up a borrowed hospital bed in their family room so Barbara could be included in the daily activity in their home. She was on oxygen most of the time, and a Dilaudid pump fed her a steady stream of pain relief.

Barbara was now quite fragile, and when she spoke it was barely a whisper, but she still loved company. I went to visit frequently, and one day following our support group session, every one of us from The Wellness Community piled into our cars and we then reconvened in Barbara's family room.

Barbara couldn't get enough information about each of us. She wanted to hear every bit of news. I marveled at her determination to remain abreast of what was happening with the other group members. Here was a woman who had every right to feel self-pity, but that never happened. At an advanced stage of illness, Barbara continued to care about others when most people wouldn't have cared about anything.

I have learned that civilians don't know how to talk to someone who is dying of cancer. Those who have danced close to death and survived, agree that family and friends above all must be honest. Don't tell the dying person that everything will be all right or that they will somehow pull through. Instead tell the person you love him or her. It is important for the dying to be surrounded by those they love, even when no words are exchanged. Don't wave hello from the doorway as if you think cancer or even imminent death is contagious. Sit on the bed and hold the person's hand.

Morrie and I had planned a Mississippi River boat cruise for the end of October. I went to see Barbara the day before we left. I took along three ice cream sundaes I'd picked up at Baskin Robbins. Barbara and I sat on her hospital bed and Roy sat on the couch nearby. We enjoyed our little ice cream party and talked about my upcoming trip.

As my departure had grown closer and Barbara had grown weaker, I'd begun to feel an overwhelming sense of uneasiness. I was fearful she might pass away while I was gone, but I never came right out and told her that I was reluctant to leave her.

When I hugged her goodbye that day she whispered in my ear, "Don't worry. I'll still be here when you return."

And she was.

I went to visit several times during the ten-day period following our return. Barbara smiled the sweetest smile every time I saw her. Her hands and feet were now swollen, but the rest of her remained painfully thin. When I hugged her, I felt her bones through the meager flesh on her back. Her cheekbones were more pronounced, and a pulse in her neck throbbed visibly; her voice was almost entirely lost. But the beauty of her soul shone through in spite of the wasted condition of her body.

Barbara never permitted the cloud of cancer to darken her disposition. In fact, a radiant glow always seemed to surround her, a fact we attributed to her belief that her death would not be an end, but rather the beginning of a peaceful existence in the hereafter. Barbara's acceptance of death made it easier for all of us. Watching her die with dignity and serenity taught me not to be afraid. Just as I'd learned from Maria, Barbara's dying taught me how to live.

On the evening of November 18, 1998, Roy was feeling depressed over Barbara's rapidly declining condition. He could tell Barbara's level of pain was on the rise, in spite of the fact that her pain medication had recently been increased. She had reached a point where she was helpless, and helplessness at the end had been her greatest fear.

The little bell that stood on her bedside table for her to summon assistance had been silent for many days. There was no way she could even lift the bell now, let alone ring it. Roy opted to spend that night in the family room rather than trying to transport Barbara into their bedroom.

Before he went to sleep, he held her in his arms and prayed for the Lord to take her that very night. He loved his wife with all his heart, but he was finally ready to let her go. He couldn't bear to see her grow any more incapacitated than she already was.

About 4:00 AM the following morning, November 19, Roy was awakened by Barbara's bell. He knew that physically she could not have picked up the bell herself, but then he also remembered that he had moved it way out of her reach. Nevertheless, the bell was ringing.

Roy got up and looked at Barbara. She looked the same. She hadn't moved. At first he couldn't bring himself to check to see whether she was still breathing. He was afraid she was dead. He was afraid that she wasn't. Finally, he did check, and Barbara was gone. She was still warm, so she hadn't been dead very long.

Roy was convinced that Barbara, or rather Barbara's spirit, had rung that bell in order to say goodbye. I agreed. Barbara would never have departed this Earth without somehow sending out a farewell message to her beloved husband.

Before her death, Barbara had planned her memorial service down to the tiniest detail. She didn't want her memorial to be a time of sorrow, but rather a celebration of faith. When Roy and Barbara planned the service with Pastor Moerer from their church, Barbara had commented that it was too bad it wasn't Easter because then she could choose the "Hallelujah Chorus" as one of her musical selections. She'd always loved that part of the Easter service, and at their church for this particular hymn, the choir would invite members of the congregation to come forward and join them. Pastor Moerer said that he thought the "Hallelujah Chorus" would be appropriate at any time of year.

But Barbara was fearful that she'd asked for too much. As a rule the choir didn't sing at memorial services, and hundreds of people would have to attend her service in order to generate the full effect this joint effort always created at Easter.

Roy asked, "If people were to find out that Barbara would like this, might it not just come about?"

The pastor answered, "It just might."

Barbara was very happy that the pastor had agreed to her request, but she was too modest to expect that people would actually go along with her idea. She had forgotten how many people respected and loved her.

When the time for the memorial was arranged, the choir members were notified and they were all eager to be there to sing for Barbara. I have never witnessed a more beautiful memorial. Close to five hundred people attended the service, and at the end the "Hallelujah Chorus" was sung. Many guests who were not regular members of the congregation joined the choir, along with congregation members, friends Barbara and Roy had known for many years. The entire front section of the church proper was lined with close to three hundred people whose voices electrified the air with this magnificent hymn.

The memorial was an awe-inspiring tribute to faith and the incredible lady who shared her faith and love with everyone she met. Barbara and I both always said that cancer was a rotten disease. But if I had to get cancer in order to meet Barbara and other remarkable people like her, then indeed cancer has hidden blessings.

Hope

Following Barbara's death, I had to face the reality that it was time for me to leave my support group family at The Wellness Community. None of my doctors would guarantee that I was "cured," but since I'd had no symptoms for close to a year, I was considered cancer-free. It wasn't fair for me to continue in the group with so many new people being diagnosed every day. Although no one was pushing me out this time, I couldn't help but feel a sense of impending loss. I also felt guilty about deserting those who remained.

Amelia Prince was still undergoing treatment for her lung cancer, living far beyond her doctor's original eighteen-month prediction, and she began to gently assure me that my leaving would be okay. I knew Amelia was right and shortly after the holidays, I told the group my decision. Ginny Baker, Arthur Schmaling, and even Amelia said they didn't want me to go, claiming I was their inspiration, but everyone rallied around me, celebrating my good health. All the wonderful people in my group would continue fighting their own individual cancer battles, and we all agreed to stay in touch.

Maryana, the group facilitator, encouraged me to sign up as an orientation volunteer at The Wellness Community, and I decided that might be an excellent way for me to repay the organization for the many services that Morrie and I had enjoyed. I received some training to learn about the various programs offered by The Wellness Community, but since I'd taken advantage of so many of these activities myself, I was almost an expert in that department to start with. By the beginning of February 1999, I was busy running orientation meetings for men and women who were new to The Wellness Community.

Most of the newcomers had been recently diagnosed, and although my job was to explain what services were available to them at The Wellness Community, I soon discovered there was something much more meaningful that I was offering these people without even realizing it.

Hope.

For the four hundred or more people who visit the Westlake Village chapter of The Wellness Community each month, hope is often the best gift one could ever give them. I remember the overwhelming fear, the terrifying thoughts that raced through my mind when I was first diagnosed. I have never felt more helpless than I did when Dr. Schilling first told me I had cancer. Newly diagnosed patients need to connect with people who have survived cancer almost as much as they need to connect with their physicians. The people I meet during these orientations figure that if I could survive cancer, perhaps they can, too. I believe that if I can make a positive difference for only one other person, all my efforts will have been worthwhile.

Many survivors feel a very strong compulsion to get on with their lives, perhaps trying to pretend their cancer never happened. Others suffer from nightmares, despair, sleep difficulties, and other disturbances similar to the Post Traumatic Stress Disorder (PTSD) experienced by survivors of war or other catastrophes.

I can fully understand the need to escape from the brutal realities of cancer, but I look at the big picture a bit differently. I believe that those of us who survive cancer and then go on to give encouragement to the newly diagnosed are contributing an essential service, support that civilians simply can't provide.

When I run my orientation groups at The Wellness Community, I promote Dr. Benjamin's books and encourage those in attendance to learn how to take part in their own recoveries. I advise anyone who has been newly diagnosed to read everything they can find about cancer and to ask questions of their physicians. It has been documented that those who read and attend support groups or workshops are more likely to survive. I tell them to surf the web, subscribe to newsletters, and talk to the survivors listed in The Wellness Community's "Buddy Book." In this marvelous resource, survivors openly write about their cancer stories and list their phone numbers for others to get in touch with them.

I want the newcomers to learn all they can about their particular cancer. I teach them that it's okay to do everything within their ability to fight back. Educating oneself brings a sense of power. Power over cancer can result when the mind-body connection is hard at work.

By February of 1999, it became apparent that Tina Rollo was losing her long, hard battle with breast cancer. She had continued making the exhaustive trips to Nashville for the vaccine she'd been receiving, but her cancer just wasn't responding to treatment of any kind.

In spite of how assiduously she had fought, Tina died on February 27. She was only 44 and left behind three beautiful young daughters, Brooke 13, Amber 11, and Megan 9.

Sometimes it just doesn't seem possible that cancer can be such a monstrous killer. When I saw Tina's husband, Tom, and her three girls at the funeral, my heart felt like a heavy stone in my chest. Tina and I should have been at a Chi Gong session, getting energized. Instead she was lying there in a coffin.

Tina's family had selected recorded music to be played over the chapel's sound system rather than live organ music, and the first song played was "My Girl" by The Temptations. Then, after a eulogy by their minister, we heard Gene Kelly's rendition of "Singing in the Rain." I don't know which song affected me more deeply, but the lyrics of both clearly symbolized what Tina was all about. She always "laughed at the clouds up above," and never lost her positive attitude. Her smile could brighten any room.

I cried almost non-stop. I cried for Tina and her three daughters; I cried for Maria and Barbara and all the others who have been so rudely taken from us because there is no cure for cancer.

I felt angry. I felt helpless.

I had to follow my heart and my instinct. There had to be some way to give more hope to <u>all</u> cancer patients. I was determined to stay active in the fight against cancer until there are no more people needing my support, no more people facing treatments that simply aren't enough to render cancer harmless.

I had joined The National Breast Cancer Coalition the previous year, but now I wanted to do more than simply read their newsletters. I filled out registration forms so Morrie and I could attend the NBCC's Seventh Annual Advocacy Training Conference scheduled to take place in Washington DC, May 22-26,1999. We were going to join the grassroots movement and "do" something about breast cancer.

As I said earlier, after a person has been declared free of active cancer, he or she will often try to put the nightmare of cancer out of mind completely. For some this may be the only way they can go on with life after enduring such a frightful experience, and I always wish these folks love and Godspeed.

But for those survivors who are able to do it, I strongly recommend working in any way possible to either support or encourage other cancer patients. I've found that running orientation meetings at The Wellness Community is wonderfully therapeutic for me, as well as advantageous to the newcomers.

Help is also especially needed in the political arena. Survivors and their loved ones can do much to raise public awareness regarding the many issues associated with cancer. Members of Congress need to know we're out here when they are called upon to vote "yea" or "nay" for funding for cancer research or health care reform legislation. We can be the deciding factor as to whether it will take continuing decades or simply a few more years to find the cure. We <u>can</u> make a difference.

The week after I signed up for the training session in Washington, I had a routine appointment scheduled with Dr. Chang. He discovered what he described as a "thickening" or small lump in my remaining breast. I forced myself to continue my positive thinking as I set up an appointment with my breast surgeon, Dr. Schilling. Because of the sneaky kind of breast cancer I'd already had, she did not think it would be prudent to attempt a needle biopsy in this instance, so she arranged a surgical biopsy for the following Monday morning.

A few hours before I went into the operating room, I sat with my stepdaughter Deborah while she did some visualization along with me. Deborah is especially gifted in her ability to create an aura of serenity. This feeling of relaxed peacefulness seems to emanate from deep within her very soul, and she wraps it around others as easily as a blanket. We summoned all the hope and healing the two of us could muster. Together we envisioned this new lump fading into nothingness.

It had been exactly one year since the "spot" in my lung had been discovered. Would I have a cancer scare on an annual basis forever more? I remembered words I'd seen printed in "Conversations!" (Cindy Melancon's ovarian cancer newsletter): "Yesterday is history. Tomorrow's a mystery. Today is a gift from God."

I had to call up every bit of hope and positive energy I possibly could. I dusted off my mantra and began repeating that no matter what this lump might be, I could beat it. I believed it. I somehow knew that this time I would indeed receive a gift from God.

And I did. This time my lump was benign.

Why Must We Beg?

Morrie and I flew to Washington, DC at the end of May for the National Breast Cancer Coalition's Seventh Annual Advocacy Training Conference. In 1991, Dr. Susan M. Love, the nation's foremost expert on breast cancer, and Philadelphia attorney Frances M. Visco, a breast cancer survivor, founded the NBCC. In 1991, two and a half million American women were living with breast cancer, and that year alone 42,000 died from the disease.

Together with a just handful of other determined women, Dr. Susan Love and Fran Visco formed the coalition, using the AIDS movement as a model. Shortly after the coalition had been created, Fran Visco was called upon to testify before an important Senate subcommittee. The very first time she spoke to this powerful group she said, "You've found billions for the benefit of white men in suits who wrecked the savings and loan industry. You found billions of dollars to fight a war in the Persian Gulf. Well, women have declared war on breast cancer and you better find a way to fund that war!"

Fran Visco and Dr. Susan Love believed that women have to do more than wear symbolic pink ribbons to fight breast cancer. They encouraged women with the disease to work together as political activists to end the breast cancer epidemic once and for all. Just eight years later, NBCC had 60,000 individual members and 500 member organizations. (http://www.natlbcc.org or contact the NBCC toll-free hotline at 1-800-622-2838)

More than 600 breast cancer survivors attended the 1999 conference and advocacy training. Forty-four states were represented, and California alone had thirty-four members in attendance. A small, but highly visible number of men joined us, and I was very proud that Morrie was one of them.

Dozens of women came up to him over the four-day period and thanked him for his support. Some of the breast cancer survivors couldn't even convince their own husbands that a conference such as this was not just for fun. (Like I've said before, the general population remains fairly ignorant when it comes to cancer.) Several of the men were there because they had lost their wives to breast cancer and we all applauded their efforts to help us.

We spent three days attending workshops, panel discussions, and plenary sessions gauged to help us understand everything from the process of drug development to the intricacies of the current leading research projects. (I'll explain the research in greater detail in the following chapter.) By educating members in the basic terms and concepts of the science involved, NBCC believed we would then be better equipped to explain NBCC legislative priorities when facing congressmen on National Lobby Day. We weren't expected to become experts, but simply to gain a foundation of scientific knowledge to empower us to be able to speak intelligently on the issues. Naturally, Morrie and I couldn't attend every session that was offered, but we tried to select from the enormous variety of topics those that seemed most interesting and timely.

From the first day, I was impressed with the thoroughness and dedication of the women in charge. The mission of NBCC is simply to eradicate breast cancer, the most common cancer among women in the United States. In order to reach this goal, NBCC trains breast cancer survivors and the friends and loved ones of women we've lost to the disease to become effective lobbyists. If a member isn't willing or able to serve as a leader, he or she is then encouraged to offer assistance to those who are leading and to be supportive of the actions taken and the decisions made on our behalf.

The bills we supported in 1999 mainly focused on legislation that would increase funding for cancer research and new laws that would ensure equal access to medical care for all women. Since its inception, NBCC has fought for and won an impressive 600 percent increase in funding for breast cancer research. The coalition was also instrumental in creating the unprecedented multi-million dollar Department of Defense (DOD) Breast Cancer Research Project in 1992. Since then NBCC support has encouraged the House and Senate to keep the DOD program active, and as a result it has attracted close to 10,000 research proposals from scientists all over the country.

For three days we attended many meetings, such as one session that focused on the controversy regarding the use of Tamoxifen as a cancer preventative. Tamoxifen, the oral chemotherapy I began taking shortly after my mastectomy, was approved in 1978 and has been used to prevent recurrence in advanced breast cancer patients. So far, it has reduced the recurrence rate by fifty percent, in spite of some disturbing side effects, such as an increased risk of uterine cancer and blood clots. Tamoxifen also causes a few less deadly problems including weight gain and a tremendous increase in hot flashes.

But the success behind Tamoxifen seems to outweigh the problems, and scientists are now testing its use as a breast cancer preventative. Moderated by Judy Woodruff, prime anchor and senior correspondent for CNN, a panel of medical experts examined the issue and answered our questions.

At subsequent workshops, foremost oncologists from all over the country explained their views, and scientists from the leading pharmaceutical companies elaborated on their long and tedious research protocol, a process necessary to get a new drug out of the laboratory and into the hands of oncologists.

One notable case study for 1999 gave us a detailed look at the growth and development of Herceptin, the very same drug that Maria Alvarez didn't receive in time. More than once during this session, I went from feeling angry to shedding tears for Maria.

Robert Bazell, panel moderator and author of Her-2: The Making of Herceptin, a Revolutionary Treatment for Breast

131

Cancer, explained the drug development procedure that was followed for Herceptin. Then panelist Dr. Susan Hellmann, Chief Medical Officer of Genentech, Inc. gave her perspective from the pharmaceutical company's point of view. We also heard from Dr. Dennis Slamon, Chief of the Division of Hematology/Oncology at UCLA; Dr. Susan Jerian, Medical Officer for the FDA; and Chris Norton, President of the Minnesota Breast Cancer Coalition. Having so many well-qualified experts in science, biotechnology, community advocacy, and government regulatory fields gave us a greater understanding of the birth of a new drug from conception to FDA approval.

At another point during our training, we were given the grim reminder that every two minutes another woman in America learns she has breast cancer. Every single day another 120 women die. We were then asked to offer a moment of silence for those NBCC members who had lost the battle with breast cancer during the past year. Photos of those who had died were projected onto a screen. Some were quite young; others looked like they could've been grandmas like me. The women were white, black, Hispanic, and Asian. Breast cancer isn't fussy about race or age.

I sent up a silent prayer for Maria and Tina. They had not lived long enough to travel to Washington to become breast cancer advocates. Both had taken journeys of a different sort. I was glad I'd been able to make the trip on their behalf. That morning I went through a whole package of tissues mopping my tears.

Some of the workshops were positively intense and I took copious notes to help me remember the vast amount of information. I was encouraged to hear that members of the scientific community, who had originally looked upon the NBCC as a nuisance, now regarded the organization as a partner.

One of the most heartening moments for the NBCC had happened the previous year at a Washington, DC social event. A scientist who works at the National Institutes of Health approached Fran Visco, NBCC's president. He told her that the National Breast Cancer Coalition had fundamentally changed the way the National Institutes of Health operates and the way their scientists now think about breast cancer. He was thrilled that NBCC had successfully lobbied for an estimated 15 percent increase in research funding for the National Institute of Health and the National Cancer Institute. For Fran his words confirmed what she already knew. The NBCC was making progress.

We finally broke into groups according to states and refined what we had learned to prepare for our visit to Capitol Hill on the last day of the conference. We organized. We networked. NBCC provided us with a voter's guide, tracking every current House and Senate member's support (co-sponsorship) on all recent legislation relating to cancer. We also received a directory of the office numbers for every legislator and a schedule listing the hours we might expect to find the representatives and senators in their offices to meet with us. The list was staggering, but Morrie and I and the other delegates from California would concentrate only on lawmakers from our home state.

By day four, May 25, 1999, we were ready to advance upon Capitol Hill. It was a marvelously clear day, not too warm, but also without any lingering clouds from the thunderstorms that had shaken the hotel earlier in the week. We assembled on the west steps of the Capitol building and heard words of encouragement from President Fran Visco and several of the NBCC board members. Chants of "Say it! Fight it! Cure it! Damn it!" echoed around the Capitol.

We rallied, we sang. One of our songs altered the words of a popular tune to: "Look Out Congress, Here We Come" and we belted it out at the top of our lungs.

Each state that was represented at the conference had a sign mounted on a long wooden pole. Our sign read: "263,000 California Women Are Living With Breast Cancer." A young man from Los Angeles whose wife had died of breast cancer carried it for us. Another sign proclaimed: "Why Must We Beg?" That one struck a chord with all of us.

The rally ended amidst tears and cheers. All the signs were collected and transported back to the hotel. Then, fueled by our enthusiasm and training, we headed directly to the halls of Congress. We went from representative to representative, explaining NBCC priorities and asking for support to enact policies that will work toward ending the breast cancer epidemic. We made it clear that we were not going to just sit back and die politely. We also dropped a few gentle reminders that breast cancer survivors are also voters who never miss an opportunity to go to the polls.

We quickly realized that we would have no more than a few minutes with each representative or senator to pitch our plea. Henry Waxman, an exceptionally competent congressman from California, walked into our meeting followed by a television camera crew. He was being taped regarding another issue even as he said hello to us and shook our hands. The camera crew left, he gave us his full attention while we spoke, pledged his support, and then immediately headed for another meeting.

Not every representative gave us as much time as Congressman Waxman. A few of our brief meetings were held while we stood in the corridors outside the congressman's office because other groups, who were also hoping to make a plea for their own causes, jammed the office's interior. We were grateful for the training we'd received because we had learned how to state our requests quickly and concisely. The NBCC had prepared handouts for us to give to the lawmakers, and I was surprised to see how extremely short and to the point these handouts were. Members of Congress, I discovered, are so overburdened with reading materials regarding legislation that the shorter the pitch, the better. We did our best to create a time-efficient opportunity to explain what research needed to be done and to request support for funding this research.

One striking insight I gained while lobbying was simply that our nation's lawmakers not only have to be convinced to help us, they have to be educated as well. We can't expect every legislator to be an expert on every bill that comes before Congress. During the previous year, the NBCC had conducted numerous Congressional Forums to educate members of Congress on breast cancer issues. NBCC had done everything in its power to assist lawmakers in creating good public policy.

But while we lobbied, clarification of the issues had to come directly from us, the individual advocates who were representing NBCC. It was up to us, for example, to explain how appropriate funding for clinical trials filters down to all cancer patients. The current monetary reimbursement from government agencies such as the National Cancer Institute given to managed care providers for patients in clinical trials is only $750 per patient. Expenses incurred by patients who participate in a trial can range as high as $6,500, so current funding falls far short of what's needed.

In another instance, we also had to point out that quality screening and treatment of breast cancer is not always available to the poor. You would think all legislators would know this, but I learned very quickly that each legislator has a personal agenda. Those who were co-sponsoring bills that related to topics such as defense or agriculture might not have taken the time to develop an extensive background in the various issues surrounding health care. We did our best to shed some light on the intricacies of health care legislation and its inherent loopholes as we explained NBCC policies and the urgency of our requests.

We made certain that every representative and senator we visited understood that we'd traveled to Washington, at our own expense, to be heard. We explained that we would all go home and vote in the next election. This may sound aggressive or even mean-spirited, but we believe that the 2.6 million women in the United States who are living with breast cancer and the one out of every eight women who will develop it in their lifetimes deserve nothing less.

I think our lawmakers got the message.

We left Capitol Hill about 6:00 PM feeling mentally exhilarated by what we had accomplished but completely exhausted otherwise. I'd learned first hand that the breast cancer battle isn't about wearing pink ribbons. As Fran Visco always says, it's about wearing <u>out</u> shoe leather.

Grab the Brass Ring

At the beginning of the twentieth century, almost no one survived cancer long term. Most lived only a few months after diagnosis. A hundred years ago cancer was indeed a death sentence. In 1971 President Richard M. Nixon asked Congress to fund research in order to find a cure for cancer. Since then, more than thirty billion dollars have been spent in the United States alone to wage war against cancer.

Today four out of every ten cancer patients are alive five years after diagnosis, so progress has definitely been made. Most of these survivors work, raise families, and enjoy productive lives, but 40 percent certainly can't be considered good enough. Chemotherapy and other drugs such as anti-nausea medications have improved dramatically in recent years, but these current developments follow decades of disappointing failures. There is still a long road ahead before we can call cancer totally curable, or ideally, preventable.

When I attended the NBCC training conference in Washington, DC, I attended sessions led by some of the foremost cancer researchers in the country. These scientists work long hours hunched over microscopes, piecing together the findings of exciting new cancer-fighting techniques that may eventually replace today's standard chemotherapy and radiation with much gentler treatments.

Techniques used to conduct research have also been on the fast track, especially in the last twenty-five years. In modern pharmaceutical laboratories, it is not unusual to find the most time-consuming and repetitious chores being performed by a robot. As a result of their persistent efforts, researchers look forward to some striking new cancer treatments in the near future.

In 1981, for example, DNA researchers identified genes within human DNA that cause cancer, and molecular biologists ultimately figured out how to reassemble genetic material, opening the door to genetically engineered microorganisms and vaccines. Since then almost every major pharmaceutical company in the U.S. has been attempting to devise procedures to identify and correct genetic errors.

These genetic mutations may be inherited or simply acquired as a result of exposure to various toxic substances in the environment. Normal cells have tumor suppressor genes that protect us from developing cancer. If these suppressor genes are damaged or mutated, cancerous cells will be able to grow. Several companies are working to develop a drug that will neutralize any destructive messages sent out by defective genes.

In the last decade alone, gene-therapy technology has realized such steady progress that scientists now seem confident that gene therapy will completely transform the treatment of cancer and many other diseases. Some form of genetic engineering could easily be the "magic bullet" that so many scientists have been seeking, eventually leading the way to a cure for cancer. The Whitehead Institute for Biomedical Research in Cambridge, Massachusetts recently reported the exciting discovery of specific genetic switches that can change a healthy human cell into a cancerous cell. By actually transforming a human cell into cancer, scientists can study how cancer spreads.

It sounds like something out of science fiction, but there is mounting evidence that someday we'll be able to alter the body's DNA, actually repairing damaged DNA, in order to find the cure. At the NBCC conference I learned that gene-therapy is already involved with human trials for the treatment of melanoma, the most aggressive form of skin cancer.

Mammograms of the future may be able to identify small spots of breast cancer that go undetected today. Diffraction-enhanced imaging or DEI, a new technique currently being developed at the U.S. Department of Energy's Brookhaven National Laboratory in New York, will use ultra-brilliant X-rays to provide a far superior contrast between normal tissue and breast tumors. Once perfected, DEI might also be used to detect tumors in other parts of the body.

Early results of an ovarian cancer research program at Cleveland Clinic Toussig Cancer Center, directed by Dr. Maurie Markman, also look very promising. According to a 1999 Ladies' Home Journal article written by Dr. Randi Hutter Epstein, Dr. Markman and his researchers have identified a chemical in the blood that has been linked to ovarian cancer. Women with ovarian cancer have higher levels of lysophosphatidic acid (LPA) in their blood, and Markman's study hopes to use this impressive discovery to identify tumors when they are small and still curable. The ability to detect ovarian tumors at the stage I level could be the most significant finding relating to women's health in the next decade.

Many studies in the area of immunotherapy have been conducted in recent years to design vaccines against cancer such as the one that Tina Rollo participated in during her visits to Nashville. Although they are available to patients in Europe, cancer vaccines are still not widely obtainable here in the U.S., except through clinical trials.

In 1998, scientists identified an immune cell capable of protecting women against breast and ovarian cancer. I know a lot of women who are praying that this stunning breakthrough will speed up the development of a breast and ovarian cancer vaccine. Encouragement for this finding comes from other parts of the world.

A vaccine called M-VAX, the first vaccine designed to fight malignant melanoma, is now being marketed in Australia. According to Business Week magazine (December 13, 1999), M-VAX is created from a combination of the patient's own melanoma cells and a special protein that permits the body's immune system to zero in on the cancer.

While we were at the conference in Washington, I also learned that the very first clinical trials for Herceptin had almost been called off because the researchers in charge of the program had difficulty signing up volunteers. The development of Herceptin probably would have been shelved indefinitely if this had actually happened. It's frightening to think that a potentially valuable drug with far-reaching benefits might never reach the public for this reason. According to Business Week (May 31,1999), prostate cancer researchers cancelled proposed trials designed to determine whether or not it would be prudent to surgically remove the prostate simply because they couldn't enroll enough patients.

As dreadful as these consequences might be, I really can't blame cancer patients for feeling reluctant to sign onto a clinical trial. The fear of being consigned to a rigid experimental protocol—much like a guinea pig—causes patients to shy away from becoming involved with the testing of new cancer treatments. A trial may save a person's life, but it is important to know there are major differences between clinical research and private medical care.

Trials are done in three phases. Phase 1 determines the maximum safe dosage of the drug along with monitoring any noxious side effects. Phase 2 investigates whether the drug works on a specific cancer. Phase 1 and 2 trials are usually conducted with a small number of patients. Phase 3 trials determine what will become standard treatment with the drug being tested. Usually the protocol for the third and final phase is a double blind study testing hundreds of patients at a time. A double blind study means that half the patients receive the drug being tested and the other half are given a placebo (sugar pill).

When one's life is precariously hanging on the line, it's scary not to know exactly what you're getting into. There is also something to be said for the psychological plus of actually "doing" something positive, and many patients with advanced stages of cancer believe that receiving a placebo just isn't enough. In a research program, the patient must be ready to accept surgery or a new drug based on the luck of the draw, just as Maria Alvarez waited for her name to be selected by a computerized lottery.

But it must be emphasized that cancer patients who volunteer for clinical trials are not only seeking a cure for their own disease but are also unselfishly paving a smoother way for future cancer sufferers. The National Cancer Institute (NCI) operates an excellent information service for the public. The NCI also coordinates a network among top cancer research and treatment centers called Cancer Information Service (CIS) that can help patients locate a potential clinical trial or other new methods of cancer treatment. (1-800-4CANCER or http://cancer.gov)

Patients can also be matched via a computer to appropriate clinical trials throughout the country. The program, called CyberMedTrials, analyzes patient data and matches it to suitable clinical trials all at no charge to the patient. (www.cybermedtrials.com)

Anti-angiogenesis drugs are also generating a lot of publicity. "Angio" refers to blood vessels in the body and "genesis" means to grow. Since cancerous tumors grow blood vessels in order to feed the cancer, the theory behind anti-angiogenesis is simply to cut off the growth of new blood vessels and literally starve the tumor to death. Ginny Benson, a retired teacher from my group at The Wellness Community who had lung cancer, first explored this avenue by traveling to a hospital in Atlanta, Georgia to take part in a trial that was experimenting with thalidomide.

Thalidomide is a mild sedative that was used by some pregnant women in the early sixties. By cutting off the blood supply to the extremities in the developing fetus, thalidomide tragically caused many babies to be born with severely underdeveloped or missing arms or legs. As soon as the relationship between thalidomide and the birth defects was discovered, the drug was taken off the market. Because of this catastrophe, the U.S. enacted legislation in 1962 that set up the stringent testing practices currently in use before a pharmaceutical product can be approved for marketing.

Years later, Thalidomide resurfaced when the anti-angiogenesis theory for cancer treatment evolved, and testing so far seems to indicate that it might be effective in treating brain tumors. If thalidomide works as a cancer treatment, it would be an unprecedented comeback for a drug that had been so unanimously condemned around the world.

Unfortunately, thalidomide in such high doses made Ginny violently ill, and she had to drop out of that program.

Subsequently, Amelia Prince and Ginny Benson became participants in the same phase 1 clinical trial for lung cancer patients at UCLA. The drug being tested is still unnamed, and the pharmaceutical company hasn't released very much information about it, but both women had some success with this trial. This new drug may prevent cancers from growing by attacking abnormal amounts of certain proteins in the blood that typically stimulate the growth of cancer cells. Along with this experimental drug, Amelia and Ginny also received approved chemotherapy regimens to help shrink their tumors.

About nine months previously, Ginny Benson's oncologist had told her that there was nothing more he could do for her. Her cancer had resisted every form of chemotherapy that he'd tried. Instead of accepting the doctor's death sentence, Ginny and her husband John took charge and sought out clinical trials that might help her. After she enrolled in this UCLA clinical trial, the fluid in her lungs disappeared and numerous small lung cancer nodules were completely annihilated.

At the time of her diagnosis, Amelia Prince was given eighteen months to live—but that was over five years ago. Her lung cancer had been considered inoperable, so Amelia received many rounds of chemotherapy before she was finally approved for participation in the same trial that Ginny Benson had discovered at UCLA.

Amelia had four tumors, but after only three months in the trial, all four tumors had shrunk a phenomenal 50 percent! This drug also cleared up the potentially damaging fluid that had collected in Amelia's lungs. Amelia has accepted that cancer has become a part of her life, but not necessarily the end of it. To a certain degree she is now able to treat her disease as a chronic illness rather than the original death sentence. When Amelia's husband Edward told me the good news about her tumor shrinkage, we both had tears of joy in our eyes.

The "Kiplinger Washington Letter" (August 6, 1999) reported that there are more than 350 new cancer drugs and vaccines currently in the development stage. Pharmaceutical companies will spend more than $1.4 billion this year alone researching new ways to combat cancer. Of course they will eventually have to go beyond experiments with laboratory rats and test these drugs on humans.

Many former clinical trial participants are alive today because they tried drugs like Carboplatin, Cytoxin, or Herceptin when they were still considered experimental. Carboplatin and Cytoxin are now used as first-line chemotherapy for many patients immediately following surgery, and Herceptin is successfully combating some forms of metastatic breast cancer. Amelia Prince and Ginny Benson, two brave women, ventured into uncharted waters to do their part in uncovering new treatment options for cancer patients.

Of course there are a lot of champions out there. Back when I was going through chemotherapy I heard from my friend Lottie Stein who lives in Palm Desert, California. She told me that her forty-year old son Randy had just been diagnosed with pancreatic cancer. Randy Stein had been advised that he had probably no more than three months to live. His family was devastated by the news, but rather than accepting the prognosis as indisputable and final, Randy sought opinions from several other oncologists. They all seemed to feel his treatment options were limited at best. He then arranged to have his surgeons send part of his tumor to the Weisenthal Cancer Group, a private cancer drug-testing laboratory in Huntington Beach, California (714-894-0011).

Researchers there assayed the cells in his tumor for sensitivity and resistance before any drugs were actually given to Randy. Clearly he didn't have time for the typical trial and error approach of chemotherapy, so his cancer's reaction to many different drugs was tested beforehand. If a particular drug didn't kill the cancer in a test tube, it was reasoned it also wouldn't kill the cancer in Randy's pancreas.

Once the assay testing had been completed, the drugs selected for Randy's chemotherapy were chemicals that normally would not have been chosen to treat pancreatic cancer. The process of quickly eliminating drugs that would have no effect at all on Randy's particular cancer led the doctors to a combination of drugs that not only had an effect, but an utterly astounding one. Four YEARS later, Randy is considered to be in complete remission.

Lottie claims Randy's recovery is a miracle, and it is, but only because Randy took matters into his own hands and played a crucial role in his own health care. He chose to fight for recovery rather than allow all responsibility for his treatment to remain in the hands of his physician. Perhaps the moral to Randy's remarkable story would be something like this: If you're ever told by a doctor that there is nothing more that can be done for you, go somewhere else!

Most oncologists shy away from these controversial assay tests—also called cancer-drug-response tests—because the procedure is still considered experimental. Oncologists tend to use drug regimens that have been duly tested over many years through closely monitored clinical trials. Many insurance plans, including Medicare, have yet to provide coverage for anything labeled experimental, so the struggle for critically ill patients to receive appropriate life-saving treatment continues.

Almost daily a new possible cure for cancer makes the news. Ginny Baker from my support group (not to be confused with Ginny Benson) entered a trial, again through UCLA, for a drug being tested for use against chronic myelogenous leukemia (CML). CML is a cancer of the bone marrow, which produces excessive numbers of immature white blood cells. Ginny's results were also amazing, and this miracle drug, later named Gleevec, is now available throughout the United States in pill form. Gleevec targets specific cancer cells, so side effects are minimal and normal healthy cells are not destroyed.

Some of the more advanced theories I've read about practically require a degree in medicine just to understand the report. The science is complex, but cancer patients can be much more hopeful today than they would have been a scant ten or fifteen years ago. Many patients with certain types of cancer who died then can now be saved.

Many sophisticated theories that are still being studied seem incredible: Scientists are actively investigating the use of tiny radioactive beads that can be implanted directly into a breast tumor, cutting treatment time to a matter of days. In the future, cancers may be frozen or vaporized with lasers. Eventually tumors will be examined with miniature fiber-optic cameras.

The long and frustrating search for a cure may have finally turned a corner. Sadly, it didn't arrive in time to save Maria Alvarez, Barbara Foerster, Tina Rollo, Ginny Benson and so many others.

I try to remember that we must apply a steady dose of positive thinking to everything that has to do with cancer. I'm thankful that many years of research have provided a cure (we must whisper the word) for Ginny Baker. I also praise dauntless fighters like Amelia Prince and Randy Stein, both initially pronounced terminal, for hanging in there long enough to grab the brass ring.

Dance Like Nobody's Watching

When I was first diagnosed I didn't think a time would ever come when I would be able to go five minutes without thinking about cancer. Cancer always seemed to occupy a niggling little spot in the back of my brain, reminding me that cancer is an all-powerful, nerve-wracking disease. I remembered how harrowing my four surgeries had been, and the brilliant red scars on my chest and abdomen helped to keep the memory always fresh in my mind. Chemotherapy had been traumatic. For a time, it seemed as if cancer had isolated me from almost everything.

Then, finally, hours would slip by when I wasn't constantly worrying about additional tumors invading my body. I gradually progressed to going days at a time without having cancer consume my every thought. Now even though my scars have faded, I can't honestly say the fear has gone away completely. I don't think about cancer constantly anymore, but it still skims in and out of my thinking. I don't think anyone who has survived cancer ever forgets the experience entirely.

I have frequent flashbacks, remembering Maria, Barbara, Tina, or Ginny, particularly when I'm enjoying a musical or theatrical performance. At a recent Hollywood Bowl concert, I thought about how Barbara would have loved being there with us, under the stars, hearing a beautiful symphony.

I wish that things could have been different for my friends who didn't make it. I miss them terribly, but I hold on to the wonderful friendships we shared, knowing that happy memories never wear out. My connection to the friends I've lost was, of course, far too brief, but I take comfort in knowing that the time we shared was truly special for them as well as for me.

My life has changed, and—aside from the loss of so many wonderful friends—surprisingly the changes are all for the better. Cancer, in its bringing one's daily routine to a sudden jolting halt, can be soul serving. Like many others who become immersed in making a living and dealing with daily problems, I'd allowed my faith to fall by the wayside.

Religion had become something I pulled up only in emergencies and on holidays, and now because of my cancer, I've reconnected—not so much with formal religion—but with God and prayer. I believe that I have gained access to immeasurable power and support through prayer, and this power is there to help me cope with anything. Nothing can happen to me that God and I can't manage together.

There are no words to properly express my gratitude to Morrie for all the loving care he lavished upon me when I was so desperately ill following my many surgeries and chemotherapy. Whenever I cried out in pain, I knew he was experiencing plenty of anguish of his own. Never once did he complain about his endless schedule of household and nursing duties. We cried together, but more often we laughed. Had Morrie not been by my side, I don't know how I would have gotten through my "cancer days."

Morrie and I are enjoying his retirement immensely. (I'm still working, writing at a leisurely pace.) Joe E. Lewis once said, "You only live once, but if you work it right, once is enough." We're doing our best to work it right. It shouldn't take a crisis like cancer to make us ease up on ourselves and take more time to enjoy one another, but sadly, it often does. Morrie and I now spend a lot of time appreciating all that we have, and we both feel very grateful that I've been given a second chance.

Being a writer, I've worked at home for years, but I now can walk away from the computer in an instant when Morrie suggests that we go for a walk or take in a movie. My work is never more important than spending time with my husband, our children, or grandchildren.

I treasure the time I spend with the grandchildren, and I look forward to each family gathering with pure joy. Briana Kiel is the oldest of our five grandchildren followed by Nancy's daughter, Maddie de Channes. Natalie Rosen and Lyla Kiel are only a few months apart in age, and the four girls now enjoy playing with our youngest grandchild, Ryan Rosen. The love of these five exquisite children was profoundly instrumental in turning the devastation of my cancer into a positive experience. They have added more to my life than I'd ever dreamed possible, constantly reminding me that my life is filled with blessings.

I've made a real effort to foster a tranquil atmosphere at home. Things get done, but much more slowly than they used to. Housework can wait. I've discovered that the world won't come to an end if I don't clean out the refrigerator. When I feel an urge to dust behind the pictures on the walls, I take a nap instead or spend the time reading or arranging loose photographs in my many photo albums.

By putting less pressure on myself to get things done, I've developed more patience with myself. This in turn has spilled over to giving me more patience with others. It's also easier these days for me to put myself in someone else's shoes, especially when I'm assisting newly diagnosed cancer patients.

Bernie Siegel is credited with saying, "You're a winner because of the way you live, not because you don't die." I am much more aware of so many things that I'd previously taken for granted. It's not as if there was no beauty in my life before cancer. Most of the time I was simply much too busy to notice. Now a radiant sunset or banks of fluffy white clouds don't ever go unnoticed. Even a clear blue sky fills me with a kind of wonder and peace.

And flowers. I'd always loved flowers and Morrie and I had worked hard to keep our garden looking presentable, but now I want to be virtually surrounded with flowers. Fortunately we live in Southern California and it's possible to find flowering plants that can be enjoyed during each season. We planted every inch of our garden with flowers, and when we ran out of space, I arranged more flowers in huge pots to brighten our patio. The flowers attract birds, especially hummingbirds, and butterflies. Our garden has been transformed into a fairyland that our grandchildren love to visit. Every time I look at the vibrant colors of my flowers dancing in the breeze, I feel blessed to be alive. Nature really does seem to have a healing influence on the mind and body, and my gardening connects me directly with that health-giving energy.

We also spend as much time as possible with our friends, especially wonderful friends like Jules and Leatrice Posner, Ruth and Allen Baker, Mary Johnson, Betty and Rick Fung and Marilyn Guild, who rallied around us when I was ill. I feel more alive when I'm linked to others. Winnie the Pooh said it best when he proclaimed, "A hug is best when shared by two."

Marilyn and her late husband Bob Guild invited us to join their Gourmet Group. The ten members of the group (including us) dine at a distinctive or unusual restaurant once a month. I also go out to lunch frequently with many other special friends such as Blandette Bush and Toni Domenic or Kit Paull and Nancy Sands, or Jonna Barr, Ruth Laage, Barbara Horne, and Judy Comford. I'm still shopping or lunching with Linda Blaustein, my friend who also survived ovarian cancer.

Knowing that it takes time to have a friend, I make an effort to stay in touch. I like to write old-fashioned letters or I pick up the phone instead of depending solely on e-mail. Each week I try to contact at least one friend I haven't connected with recently. I want to maintain my friendships with all the caring people who have touched my life over the years.

I don't expect that doing the little things I enjoy most will necessarily extend my life by decades, but certainly by one lovely day at a time. By trying to "live" more fully and to nurture my human connections, I feel I've grown as a person.

At least once a year, we try to travel to a place we've never visited before such as our trip to Scotland with Betty and John. I will never forget the impact of my sudden spiritual awareness at Iona Abbey. Did the Scottish saints actually guide me, or was it simply time for me to gather strength on my own?

The following year we toured the waterways of Russia, the birthplace of Morrie's mother, with friends Anne and Jerry Olivarez. We also visited Sweden, and we experienced an unforgettable journey through Alaska with Ruth and Allen Baker.

We've taken a leisurely steamboat trip up the Mississippi River with our friend Gertrude Pomish and we spent another week getting to know the delightful town of Savannah, Georgia with Joan and Barney Barco. Along the way, we've met many interesting people, and we've seen extraordinary sights. At the moment we have plans to visit China, Tibet, and Bali, and we're hoping we'll be able to travel wherever our dreams take us for many more years to come.

I also try to spend some quiet time alone. I've learned not to feel guilty when I devote an entire day to reading or indulging myself in some other fashion. I seldom watch more than an hour of TV per day, and many days I skip it completely. I allow myself to relax. I try to find time each day to take ten or twenty deep, unhurried breaths to release any tensions that may have crept into my body. This is not to say that I don't occasionally get stressed or uptight. I do. But I am now more centered in such a way that little things don't do me in completely as they may have in the past.

I am always thrilled when I read about cancer survivors achieving surprising goals. A cancer survivor who wins the Grand Prix or a group of breast cancer survivors who attempt to scale the slopes of Mt. McKinley in Alaska are clearly battling more than the rigors of a grueling bicycle race or the challenge of climbing the highest peak in North America.

<u>Friendly Exchange</u> magazine recently ran an article by Erika Schutz telling how a team of women, including five breast cancer survivors, tried to fight their way to the top of

Mt. McKinley. Foul weather kept them from reaching the actual summit, but it didn't stop them from filming a ninety-minute documentary about their adventure. Their production of "Climb Against the Odds" was created in order to increase breast cancer awareness, but it's also a glorious success story that is a lesson in fortitude and determination for all of us.

Six months after my first experience as a lobbyist for breast cancer funding, I learned the results of our efforts. The 106th Congress appropriated the full $175 million for the Department of Defense Breast Cancer Research Program that the National Breast Cancer Coalition had requested. This was $40 million more than the previous year's funding! NBCC also succeeded in getting Congress to provide more funds for breast cancer research at the National Institutes of Health in Washington.

No, the many courageous members of the NBCC who are waging war against breast cancer haven't changed the world, at least not yet. But just give us time.

We will continue to urge Congress to support research and improved treatment options. We will let the politicians know that women are no longer willing to simply wear pink ribbons to show their support for the fight against breast cancer. Instead we want to see green dollars funded by our lawmakers in Washington. We want to end this epidemic forever.

Cancer isn't supposed to have positive, far-reaching benefits, but through my contacts with The Wellness Community, the Ovarian Cancer National Alliance, the National Breast Cancer Coalition, and the American Cancer Society, I've discovered that I'm not the only survivor who feels something good has resulted from an experience with cancer.

I am especially grateful for the love and friendship of all the terrific people I met at The Wellness Community. I will never forget the strength and courage of those who survived and especially of those who didn't. The faith, love, and spiritual insights of my cancer "buddies" continue to inspire me.

We discovered that life is not fair, but by reaching out to one another we were able to stand tough against a very frightening disease. There was a certain kind of magic in learning we were not alone. We erased the fear by touching each other's hearts and souls.

Just look at me.

I am alive.

What do I do, now that I've survived cancer?

I exercise.

I replace my toothbrush often, (though not every seventy-two hours).

I take pleasure in nature, and I take care to recycle.

I listen to my favorite music. I listen to Dr. Laura on the radio.

I continue to learn everything I can about cancer so I can be an educated advocate. I work toward doing my share to eradicate all cancers, especially breast and ovarian.

I've learned that I still have a lot to learn.

I constantly rejoice in my good fortune and in the magic of healing.

I've learned that the most important thing in life is to love. The second most important is sharing that love.

Each day I try to think of one thing for which I can be grateful and I thank God.

I've learned that if I don't want to snap like a twig, I must bend a little.

I know that I have to let go of all the trivial problems in my life in order to have the strength to deal with the important ones.

I now see my life as a journey, and I can change the direction of my travel whenever I choose. It's all up to me. I can even look within myself and change my attitudes.

I will reach out to people with cancer and try to inspire them to remember that as long as they are alive, there is hope.

I've learned that the fear of a cancer recurrence is always there, but I don't have to accept that fear. I can face it down.

I've learned that life is tough, but I'm tougher.

I've learned to enjoy life in whatever way I choose and not worry about what others may think.

I now know that it's okay for a grandma to let loose and do the Charleston, the jitterbug, or even the twist.

And when I dance, I dance like nobody's watching.

RESOURCES

American Cancer Society, 1599 Clifton Road, NE, Atlanta, GA 30329-4251. 1-800-ACS-2345. http://www.cancer.org

Anti-Cancer, Inc., (chemotherapy-sensitivity testing) 7919 Ostrow Street, San Diego, CA 92111. 619-654-2555, fax 619-268-4175. http://www.anticancer.com

CancerCare, Inc. 800-813-4673. http://www.womenintheknow.com

"Conversations!" The International Newsletter for Those Fighting Ovarian Cancer. Editor: Cindy H. Melancon, PO Box 7948, Amarillo, TX 79114-7948. 806-355-2565. http://www.ovarian-news.com

"Coping with Cancer" Magazine. Media America, PO Box 682268, Franklin, TN 37068. 615-790-2400.

CyberMedTrials, (matches patient with clinical trials) http://www.cybermedtrials.com

National Breast Cancer Coalition, 1707 L Street NW, Suite 1060, Washington, DC 20036. 202-296-7477, fax 202-265-6854. http://www.stopbreastcancer.org

National Cancer Institute (NCI) Cancer Information Service (CIS), Bethesda, MD 20892.
Hotline:1-800-4-CANCER or 1-800-422-6237. For information regarding clinical trials: http://cancer.gov or http://cancertrials.nci.nih.gov.

National Ovarian Cancer Coalition, 2335 East Atlantic Boulevard, Suite 401, Pompano Beach, FL 33062. 888-OVARIAN. http://www.ovarian.org

Ovarian Cancer National Alliance (OCNA), 1627 K Street, NW, 12th Floor, Washington, DC 20006. 202-331-1332. http://www.ovariancancer.org

Reach to Recovery (for breast cancer patients). Contact the American Cancer Society (above).

Weisenthal Cancer Group, (chemotherapy-sensitivity testing) 15140 Transistor Lane, Huntington Beach, CA 92649. 714-894-0011, FAX 714-893-3658.

The Wellness Community, 2716 Ocean Park Blvd., Santa Monica, CA 90405-5211. 310-314-2555, fax 310-314-7586.

Women's Cancer Network: http://www.wcn.org

BIBLIOGRAPHY

Arnst, Catherine, "The War Against Cancer Needs New Recruits," <u>Business Week</u>, May 31, 1999, p. 50.

Bazell, Robert, <u>Her-2: The Making of Herceptin, a Revolutionary Treatment for Breast Cancer</u>, Random House, New York, 1998.

Benjamin, Harold H., <u>The Wellness Community Guide to Fighting for Recovery from Cancer</u>, G. P. Putnam's Sons, New York, 1995.

Epstein, Randi Hutter, "The Top 10 Researchers in Women's Health, <u>Ladies' Home Journal</u>, March 1999, pp. 88-90.

Ferre, Julia, <u>Basic Macrobiotic Cooking</u>, George Ohsawa Macrobiotic Foundation, Oroville, CA, 1987.

Hirshberg, Caryle and Barasch, Marc Ian, <u>Remarkable Recovery</u>, Riverhead Books, New York, 1995.

_____ "The Kiplinger Washington Letter," Washington, DC, August 6, 1999, p. 2.

Licking, Ellen, Editor, "Teaching the Body to Fight Cancer," <u>Business Week</u>, December 13, 1999, p. 117.

Love, Susan M. with Lindsey, Karen, <u>Dr. Susan Love's Breast Book</u>, Addison-Wesley Publishing Co., Reading, Massachusetts, 1991.

Piver, M. Steven with Wilder, Gene, <u>Gilda's Disease</u>, Prometheus Books, Amherst, New York, 1996.

Radner, Gilda, It's Always Something, Avon Books, New York, 1989.

Schutz, Erika, "Fighting the Odds," Friendly Exchange, C-E Publishing, Warren, Michigan, Fall 1999, pp. 12-20.

Sears, Barry with Lawren, Bill, The Zone, Regan Books, Harper-Collins, New York, 1995.

Simonton, O. Carl, et. al., Getting Well Again, Bantam Books, New York, 1992.

Spiegel, David, Living Beyond Limits: New Hope and Help for Facing Life-Threatening Illness, Fawcett Books, New York, 1994.

Weil, Andrew, Spontaneous Healing, Alfred A. Knopf, New York, 1995.

Additional Suggested Readings

Benjamin, Harold H., From Victim to Victor, Jeremy P. Tarcher, Inc., Los Angeles, 1987.

Joyce, Marilyn, 5 Minutes to Health, published by 5 Minutes to Health, Los Angeles, CA, 1995.

Kaye, Ronnie, Spinning Straw into Gold, Simon & Schuster, Inc., New York, 1991.

Keane, Maureen and Chace, Daniella, What to Eat If You Have Cancer, Contemporary Books, Inc., Chicago, 1996.

Link, John, The Breast Cancer Survival Manual, Henry Holt and Company, New York, 1998.

Siegel, Bernie S., Love, Medicine & Miracles, HarperCollins Publishers, New York, 1986.

Virag, Irene, We're All in This Together, Andrews and McMeel, Kansas City, Missouri, 1995.

Weil, Andrew, Eight Weeks to Optimum Health, Alfred A Knopf, New York, 1997.

Cassette Tapes

"Chemotherapy," read by the author, Belleruth Naparstek, Time Warner Audio Books, Los Angeles, 1993.

"Getting Well," read by the author, O. Carl Simonton, M.D., Audio Renaissance Tapes, Inc., Los Angeles, 1987.

"Love Medicine and Miracles," read by the author, Bernie S. Siegel, M.D., Harper Audio, HarperCollins Publishers, Inc., 1988.

"Relaxation and Guided Imagery," read by the author, Harold H. Benjamin for use by participants of The Wellness Community.

"Visualization: Directing the Movies of Your Mind," by Adelaide Bry, read by Julie Just, Audio Renaissance Tapes, Inc., Los Angeles, 1989.